TECHNOLOGY AND IN/EQUALITY

Questioning the information society

Edited by
Sally Wyatt, Flis Henwood,
Nod Miller and Peter Senker

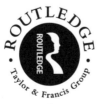

London and New York

First published 2000
by Routledge
11 New Fetter Lane, London EC4P 4EE

Simultaneously published in the USA and Canada
by Routledge
29 West 35th Street, New York, NY 10001

Typeset in 10/12pt Sabon by
The Midlands Book Typesetting Company Ltd
Printed in Great Britain by
TJ International Ltd, Padstow, Cornwall

British Library Cataloguing in Publication Data
A catalogue record for this book is available
from the British Library

Library of Congress Cataloguing in Publication Data
Sally Wyatt, Flis Henwood, Nod Miller and Peter Senker

ISBN 0-415-23023-3 (pbk)
ISBN 0-415-23022-5 (hbk)

CONTENTS

FIGURES

TABLES

PREFACE

All the contributors to this book are based in, or have close associations with, the Department of Innovation Studies in the University of East London, which promotes an interdisciplinary approach to learning, teaching and research about new technologies, science and society. Theoretical orientations, disciplines and fields of specialism represented in this book range across computer science, physics, sociology, science, technology and society studies (STS), economics, women's studies, history, adult education and media and cultural studies. We believe that this breadth of perspectives is a strength, and each of us has learned a good deal from the insights which arise from conversations across the boundaries between disciplines. In the course of putting this book together, there have been times when we have struggled to understand each other's language and assumptions, but engaging in these struggles has often yielded new insights about aspects of the world which we had taken for granted. We hope that this book will stimulate similar reflections of unquestioned realities amongst its readers.

The Editors

ACKNOWLEDGEMENTS

We are indebted to all our colleagues in the Department of Innovation Studies, past and present, for their help and support in developing the ideas explored in this book, and for their commitment to addressing issues of in/equality in their professional practice. Gill Perkins deserves our particular gratitude for her patience and painstaking attention to detail in the preparation of the manuscript for publication.

We should also like to thank the following friends and colleagues, for stimulating debates, challenging and constructive comments, and practical help in putting this book together: Alison Adam, Rod Allen, Ellen Balka, Wiebe Bijker, Michael Cardona, Helen Fairlie, Gill Kirkup, David Morley, Dave O'Reilly, Hazel Platzer, Hans Radder, Cath Senker, Jacky Senker, Jackie Stacey, Liz Stanley and Andrew Webster.

We are grateful to Carlota Perez for permission to use Figure 8.1; and to Macmillan Ltd. for permission to use material from P. Bairoch and M. Levy-Loboyen (eds) *Disparities in Economic Development since the Industrial Revolution* (1981) in Table 8.3.

Sally, Flis, Nod and Peter
(Amsterdam, Brighton, London and Brighton)

CONTRIBUTORS

All contributors are members of the Department of Innovation Studies, UEL, unless otherwise indicated.

Rod Allen is Head of the Department of Journalism at City University, London. In earlier lives he was a magazine editor and publisher, a television current affairs producer, a broadcasting executive, a multimedia consultant and a computer geek.

Chris Freeman is Emeritus Professor at the University of Sussex and a Visiting Professor in the Department of Innovation Studies. He was formerly Director of the Science Policy Research Unit (SPRU), University of Sussex. His most recent publications include books with Luc Soete on *Mass Unemployment and Computerised Technical Change* and *The Economics of Industrial Innovation*.

Flis Henwood undertakes research in the field of gender, science and technology and is interested in questions of culture and identity in educational and work settings.

Helen Kennedy is a senior lecturer in multimedia studies at the University of East London. She was previously a tutor/ researcher on Project @THENE.

Linda Leung was a tutor/researcher on Project @THENE and a lecturer in multimedia studies. Currently, she is completing her PhD, entitled 'Where Am I? Locating Self and Ethnicity on the WWW'. She has previously taught and/or conducted research at the Universities of London, North London, Miami and Western Sydney.

Nod Miller is Professor of Innovation Studies and Assistant Vice-Chancellor (Lifelong Learning) at UEL. Her perspectives on technology and in/equality are informed by her working class origins and her enthusiasm for popular television as well as by her professional identities as sociologist and adult educator.

Alvaro de Miranda recently retired as Head of the Department. He is a former President of the European Inter-University Association on Society, Science and Technology. He is currently working on a Lifelong Learning project in association with trade unions.

Herbert Pimlott has worked in professional and alternative media. He has taught communication and cultural studies at the Universities of North London and East London, Middlesex University and Goldsmiths' College. He now teaches communication studies at the University of Windsor in Canada.

Sarah Plumeridge conducted research for her MPhil exploring the pedagogic construction of gender and technology discourses within an undergraduate context.

Gavin Poynter is Head of the Department of Innovation Studies and has recently completed a book entitled *Restructuring in the Service Industries, management reform and workplace relations in the UK service sector* published by Cassell in 2000.

Peter Senker is a Visiting Professor in the Department, an Honorary Fellow of SPRU and Chair of IPRA Ltd, a network company which researches training and Information Technology. He has studied social and economic implications of technological change since 1972.

Linda Stepulevage is a senior lecturer in the Department. Her research explores women's relationship to computing and the development of technical skills and knowledge. She is especially interested in how sexuality, 'race' and class inform these relations.

Graham Thomas has carried out policy research on the development of telematic services in the UK and Europe. He is also active as a user representative in the UK Internet community.

Kathy Walker's research interests include the development and application of new communication technologies, their implications for issues of access to and control of the media, and their impact on public service broadcasting.

Sally Wyatt is a Reader in the Department of Innovation Studies, though she is currently based at the University of Amsterdam. She has never owned a car and she does not regard this as deprivation.

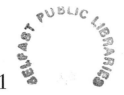

1

CRITICAL PERSPECTIVES ON TECHNOLOGIES, IN/EQUALITIES AND THE INFORMATION SOCIETY

Flis Henwood, Sally Wyatt, Nod Miller and Peter Senker

In October 1999, *The Guardian* reported that the British Prime Minister Tony Blair was about to 'take his first tentative steps into information technology' (*The Guardian* 25 October 1999: 8). He admitted his incompetence in the face of a computer, and attended a two-hour training session in a shopping centre to be instructed in word-processing, e-mail and the Internet. This was part of a publicity drive to encourage people to get involved in technology through a network of e-libraries. *The Guardian* accompanied its report of Blair's introduction to IT training with an article by the Prime Minister in which he marvelled at the 'speed of change of the new industrial revolution sweeping the world'. He asserted that the future of the nation was dependent upon technological success, arguing that computers and the Internet were powering economic growth, and that ensuring Britain was not divided into computer haves and have-nots was fundamental to the building of a fair as well as a prosperous society.

The story of the Prime Minister's recent encounters with technology illustrates neatly some of the themes and preoccupations of this book. Our intention is to provide critical perspectives on the relationships between information and communication technologies (ICTs) and the social and economic structures and processes which affect equality and inequality. Blair apparently views computers as magical entities with the power to transform society,

1

and this perspective exemplifies the assumptions underlying much policy thinking. Contributors to this book challenge this policy rhetoric, question the assumption that there is a straightforward causal connection between technology and socio-economic progress, and suggest that the extremes of utopian or dystopian thinking about technology do not stand up to scrutiny.

The fact that Blair is ignorant about the use of information technologies illustrates one aspect of the complexity of the issues at play here. He makes reference to the division between computer haves and have-nots, and to the need for IT centres to be established in 'the poorest parts of the country' as if there were a necessary connection between poverty and ignorance. This is ironic, as he himself possesses considerable power and is relatively prosperous, but had not previously engaged directly with ICTs. Rich, powerful people seem to have something in common with the very poor: members of the British royal family, like homeless people, rarely carry cash; senior executives of large companies, in common with Tony Blair, often live in ignorance of commonplace office technologies, since they generally have secretaries who receive and print out their e-mail. Like people who cannot afford to buy computers, many of the rich and powerful lack access to computers, or to the knowledge required to use them. Such contradictions are among the themes dealt with in the chapters which follow.

We share the Prime Minister's belief in the importance of engaging with technologies and taking them seriously, but we question the assumption that there are simple technological fixes to complex social problems. In this book we bring critical perspectives to bear on the use of terms such as 'the information society' and explore contrasting views of the way in which inequality in relation to technology is conceptualised. We have chosen to use the term 'in/equality' in the title of this book because we believe it is important to recognise that the concept of inequality necessarily implies a concept of equality, and *vice versa*. The slash (/) is useful in reminding us of the need to keep in mind the relative nature of equalities and inequalities in relation to technological objects and processes, and of the need to avoid the utopian/dystopian polarisation which often features in debates about technological and social change.

Contributors to the book were asked to use the terms equality and inequality critically, to make explicit the ways in which the issues discussed relate to the subject of technology and in/equality, to specify which particular in/equalities were being addressed in their chapters, and to demonstrate how analysis of their empirical data can further understanding of the relationship between technology and in/equality.

THE AIMS OF THIS BOOK

The key questions framing this book are:

- What are the theoretical and policy implications of questioning the 'information society' and the widely-held assumption that more technology and/or information is better?
- Why is it important to think about technology and in/equality?
- Is it possible and/or desirable to move away from a universalist notion of equality to one that is situated and contextualised?
- What theoretical ideas can help us to understand technology and in/equality?
- How can we use past experiences to inform current debates about new technological developments?

The rest of this chapter sets the scene for the exploration of these questions by locating our approach in relation to previous debates about technology and inequality. We explore the concept of inequality and explain our position in relation to what we believe to be an unnecessarily polarised division in the social sciences between those analyses which focus on structures of inequality and those which are concerned with the experience and meaning of inequality at the level of the individual. We examine contrasting ways in which the technology-society relationship is characterised in the literature on science, technology and society (STS). We offer a critique of the concept of the 'information society' and conclude with a sketch of the organisation of the rest of the book.

WHY INEQUALITY?

New information and communication technologies feature prominently in public discussions about the potential for people to be liberated from the constraints imposed by their bodies or by geography. We aim to contribute to theoretical and policy debates about the place of ICTs in society and to promote dialogue amongst scholars and practitioners across a variety of disciplines and fields of practice. In particular, we wish to intervene in the debate about the 'information society' by questioning some of the assumptions made concerning the relationship between technological change and economic, social and cultural change.

Many 'information society' enthusiasts, both academics and policymakers, claim that the use of ICTs will relieve people of drudgery, improve access to information and entertainment, and result in greater social justice. Dissident voices suggest that the application of ICTs will exacerbate social inequalities through the creation of information haves and have-nots, result in greater social control through the growth of electronic surveillance and polarise the labour market. Technological determinism can be detected on both sides of this polarised debate. We seek to analyse both the potentials and constraints represented by technologies in specific contexts. We focus on applications of ICTs in the media industries, in education and in work because of their position in respect of access to and control over crucial resources such as information, knowledge, skills and income. Some of the key issues addressed include: democracy and broadcasting technologies; gender, class and ethnicity in technological education and lifelong learning; class, gender and skills in the workplace; and the global economic inequalities associated with technological innovation.

Many of the chapters in this book incorporate historical perspectives, examining past and present technologies in order to illustrate the dissonance between promises of emancipation and the reality of the ways in which new technologies are distributed and controlled. Contributors seek to further theoretical understanding of the relationship between technology and inequality by questioning the meanings of these terms and by challenging the widespread association of technology with progress.

Several conceptual and theoretical issues concerning our definition and use of the terms equality and inequality should be clarified at this point. We have to ask 'equality of what, and for whom?' Equality is often judged by comparing one particular aspect of an individual, such as income, wealth, health, happiness or education with the same aspect of another. Amartya Sen, winner of the Nobel Prize for economics in 1998, points out that,

> [e]quality in terms of one variable may not coincide with equality in another. For example, equal opportunities can lead to very unequal incomes. Equal incomes can go with very significant differences in wealth. Equal wealth can coexist with very unequal happiness.
>
> (Sen 1992: 2)

We do not understand inequality to be the same as deprivation, although the two may coexist. Deprivation may be absolute and/or universal, while inequality is always relative. Neither do we understand inequality to be simply about differences in the possession of, or access to, goods, services and attributes. Such differences and diversity do not necessarily imply inequality. Difference and diversity are, however, prerequisites for inequality where the lack of goods, services or attributes confers an actual and/or perceived disadvantage.

For there to be inequality, there have to be both difference and disadvantage. For this reason, the contributors to this book do not simply point out differences which relate to technology – for example, differential access to the Internet – but they also try to explore how, and explain why, such differences also constitute disadvantages. Furthermore, disadvantage and inequality are both relative terms, and so the question of which individuals or groups are disadvantaged and in relation to which others is also a central theme running throughout the book.

It is also useful to look at issues of inequality from a global economic perspective. For more than two hundred years, economists have been striving to understand the creation of wealth and income. The distribution of the benefits (and costs) of economic growth has received much less attention from mainstream economists, who have largely been preoccupied with the growth of variables such as employment and national income. Development economics, however, now embraces the Human Development Index (HDI), which is not exclusively focused on economic opulence as GNP is. This index, which is used in recent United Nations *Human Development Reports*, is based on three distinct components – indicators of longevity, education and income per head. The HDI attempts to capture in 'one single number a complex reality about human development and deprivation' (Sen 1999: 23). The most recent United Nations *Human Development Report* points out that although the world has become much more prosperous in the last fifty years, the numbers of people who have incomes of less than one dollar a day, who lack access to clean water, and who die before they reach forty years of age each exceeds one billion. More than 800 million people are malnourished (UNDP 1999). These statistics illustrate the very real levels of deprivation which continue to exist in the provision of the most basic facilities.

We have already suggested the importance of acknowledging the significance of perception in relation to inequality and disadvantage. Different people, and different groups of people, have different goals and value systems. As Sen argues, 'the ethics of equality has to take adequate note of our pervasive diversities' (1992: 28). Some 'poor' people may be happy with their lot. Others in similar economic circumstances may be discontented as a result of comparing themselves with those who are marginally better off than themselves. Marginal improvements may be seen as attainable whereas the lifestyles of those significantly richer may be seen as so different as to be unimaginable. Poverty is sometimes proclaimed to be a virtue, although it is noticeable that such virtue is advocated by those who do not suffer from it themselves (Tawney 1964).

Despite variations in perception, within individual societies there is usually some kind of consensus about which social and economic goods are important and which, if unequally distributed, would contribute most towards economic and social inequality. Maslow (1962) saw the motives underlying behaviour as being patterned in terms of what he called a 'hierarchy of needs' and argued that people will only strive to fulfil needs higher up the ladder when those lower down have already been fulfilled; he postulated a set of five needs, ranging from biological survival needs as the most basic, through the needs for safety, affiliation or belonging, and self-esteem, to the need for 'self-actualisation', or achievement of one's full potential. This might be translated into a hierarchy of goods and services, with the most basic being food, clothing and shelter; social goods such as safety, health care, education, transport and communications rank next in importance. Over time, the composition of the hierarchy changes: car ownership would not have featured on a list of key indicators of inequality a century ago. Yet today, access to and ownership of telephones, television, home computers and Internet accounts are all seen as indicators of inequality within and between social groups. The contributors to this book are particularly concerned to understand in which specific historical, social and cultural contexts differential access to, and control over, new technologies become constituted as inequalities.

In order to address this question, contributors have utilised theoretical frameworks which emphasise both the material and the symbolic aspects of inequality. Research in the social sciences has a long tradition of identifying and examining the economic and social inequalities associated with the collectivities of class, gender and ethnicity. Such research has sought to identify the material disadvantages experienced by particular social groups and the structures within which these inequalities are reproduced. However, more recently, social theorists who adopt postmodernist approaches have moved away from the analysis of social structures to a study of social meanings and the way in which these are embodied in culture. Postmodernists have also been less concerned with the categories of class, gender and ethnicity and more interested in identities, subjectivities and individual agency. We occupy the middle ground in what we see as a false dichotomy between structure and individual agency. Following Giddens, whose 'theory of structuration' (1976; 1984) seeks to overcome the dualism of structure and action, we seek to integrate the analysis of structures with actors and meanings.

In her study of inequality, Bradley (1996), too, follows Giddens in attempting to integrate structure and agency. However, she argues that the term 'structure' may be inappropriate in that it over-emphasises stasis in social relations. She argues that social relationships are constantly evolving and highlights the interaction of what she calls 'the two faces of social reality: ... continuity within change, order within variability, fixity within fluidity' (1996: 7). Bradley goes on to argue that 'there is no contradiction between seeing social phenomena as social constructs and seeing them as objectively lived relationships, so long as the mutual and circular relationship between the two aspects is acknowledged' (1996: 8).

A further important point about our understanding of inequality is that it is also about power. Again, both material and symbolic aspects are important here. Thus, as Bradley has argued, while symbolic aspects of power, such as those highlighted in discourse theory, are extremely important, they constitute only one dimension of the power relations which are embodied in social inequalities (1996: 9). To illustrate this point, we might consider gendered power relations. Men may be able to disempower women by marginalising them in dominant discourse; and women, through the redefinition and the rewriting of discourses, may be able to relocate themselves at the centre or empower themselves in a symbolic sense. However, it is only when material resources are moved in alignment with such discourses that it becomes possible to identify the relatively more and less advantaged or powerful groups. It is when the differences in the material positions of men and women brought about through processes such as marginalisation, exclusion or segregation constitute a disadvantage to either group that it becomes legitimate to talk about gender inequality.

The contributions to this book deal in varying ways with Bradley's 'two faces of social reality'. They address the individual and/or collective actions that shape the direction and experience of technological change as well as the social, economic, cultural and technological factors that act to constrain, structure and shape those actions. Some contributors are particularly concerned with the development or experience of technologies at the material level, as in the chapters by Chris Freeman and Peter Senker which focus on the global economic and social inequalities associated with technological change. Other contributors are more concerned with understanding the symbolic significance of particular technologies and associated skills and knowledges and with the experience of inequality at the local level. The chapter by Nod Miller, Helen Kennedy and Linda Leung and the one by Flis Henwood, Sarah Plumeridge and Linda Stepulevage on education are examples of such an approach. Our intention is to explore the relationship between the material and the symbolic in order to throw light on the nature and experience of inequalities that are associated with the development and implementation of ICTs. In this way, we aim to produce analyses that are situated both historically and culturally. Before going on to discuss how technology and inequality have been addressed in the information society literature to date, we briefly review the different ways in which the technology-society relationship has been understood in the STS literature.

RELATIONSHIPS BETWEEN TECHNOLOGY AND SOCIETY[1]

There are three main ways in which relationships between technological change and social change are understood in popular debate and academic literature. The first is 'technological determinism', in which technologies emerge as if from nowhere and then proceed to transform the society into which they are diffused. A second perspective, which may be summed up as 'technology as neutral', also has the technology emerging from nowhere but, in this perspective, the implication is that people choose how they want to use it. The third perspective, 'constructivism', emphasises the origins and development of technology, demonstrating how people are involved in the creation of technical networks, not only in how they are subsequently used.

The habit of thought and language of ascribing simple cause and effect to relationships between technology and society is pervasive. The following are examples of statements commonly made about the 'effects' of various technologies:

- In the twentieth century, the car became widely available, leading Americans to move to the suburbs and providing a symbol of freedom reflected in many American road movies, books and songs.
- The invention of television caused the decline of the cinema and a deterioration of children's reading abilities.
- The development of the contraceptive pill resulted in the sexual permissiveness of the 1960s and a reduction of family size.

Thinking about relationships between technology and society in terms of effects has been 'common sense' for so long that it has not needed a label. But its critics have termed it technological determinism. This approach is usually associated with the notion that technological progress represents social progress.[2] It suggests that each generation produces a few inventors, whose inventions appear to be both the determinants and stepping stones of human development. Unsuccessful inventions are condemned by their failure to the dustheap of history. Successful ones soon prove their value and are rapidly integrated into society, which they proceed to transform. In this sense, a technological breakthrough is claimed to have important social consequences. This view pervades the 'information society' literature discussed below.

The simplicity of this model is a principal reason for its endurance. But it is also the model which makes most sense of many people's experience. For most people, most of the time, the technologies they use every day are of mysterious origin and design. Most people have no idea from whence the technologies came and equally little idea of how they actually work. People simply adapt themselves to their requirements and hope that they continue to function in the predictable and expected ways promised by those who sold them. It is because technological determinism conforms with a majority of people's experience that it remains the 'common sense' explanation.

The problem with technological determinism is that it leaves no space for human choice or intervention and, moreover, absolves people from responsibility for the technologies they make and use. This serves the interests of those responsible for developing new technologies, regardless of whether they are consumer products or power stations. Technological determinism allows people to deny responsibility for the technological choices they make individually and collectively, and to ridicule those people who do challenge the pace and direction of technological change. At the very least, there are choices about the use of technologies, and if people choose to use them, they also have choices about how they do so. This is the starting point for the notion of 'technology as neutral', in which the origins of technologies are not problematised but the ways in which they are used most certainly are.

The conception of technology as a neutral instrument which people can use as they wish challenges the claim of technological determinism that technologies have straightforward social effects. This explanation is far too simple, given the wide variety of situations in which technologies are introduced. The advantage of the 'technology as neutral' model over technological determinism is that it gives a prominent place to people, individually and in groups, making choices about how they want to use technical arte-facts. Technological determinism allows no room at all for what is usually a very messy process of change, involving not only new technical artefacts but also a range of broadly social factors, including struggles over political, economic and cultural control within and between countries, organisations and households. 'Technology as neutral' begins to create a space in which complex and usually conflict-ridden historical processes can be explored. Investigation of that space, however, soon reveals that the proc-esses by which technologies themselves are created are just as riven with choice and conflict as any other historical process. In other words, the first part of technological determinism, that technolo-gies simply follow an internal, technical logic free of social forces, also requires closer examination. Such examination will begin to reveal the limits of the 'technology as neutral' approach.

The essence of the constructivist argument is that technologies are objects made by people. They are not separate from but rather are constituted by political, economic and cultural processes. Looking closely at any technology will reveal that it is marked by the conditions of its design, production and use. Whereas techno-logical determinism presents social change as being the result of technological change, social constructivism explains technologies as being actively shaped by different social groups. Moreover,

10

social constructivism sometimes regards the distinction between society and technology as an arbitrary one, if sometimes an analytically and practically useful distinction.

There are three ways in which technologies can be said to be social constructions:

- technologies are the material embodiment of the values and interests of particular social groups or classes;
- cultural meanings of technologies are elements in language and in symbolic universes; and,
- the workings of technologies are the outcome of negotiation between individuals, groups and institutions.

According to the first proposition, things, machines and technologies are not just things, machines and technologies that perform useful functions. They are also ideas made real. Designers, engineers and their managers and financiers have values, goals, assumptions and even prejudices that are built into technologies. For example, the predominant design of cars presupposes the existence of nuclear families. This is sometimes referred to as the 'social shaping of technology' approach (MacKenzie and Wajcman 1985).

The second proposition is informed by the work of Pierre Bourdieu (1984). Here, the social and cultural meanings given to technical artefacts through the processes of consumption or use are emphasised. A car is not simply an internal combustion engine with seats and a radio in a steel casing on wheels. Whether or not people own cars at all and, if they do, their makes, ages and colours all provide meaning for them and others about who they are and what their values and aspirations are. This is not only the case for individuals; production technologies used by companies indicate to their competitors something about their commitment to modernisation and about their attitude to their workers. At a national level, weapons systems are not merely collections of warheads and missile launchers; they provide a country with a sense of prestige and give signals to other nations about intentions and capabilities. Here, technologies are not primarily material objects but constitute an arena for contesting meaning. The physical capabilities of the artefacts are not paramount; rather the cultural meanings given to them or read into them are important. Because these meanings are contested and fought over by different social groups, the same artefact will be understood differently over time and across cultures.

The third type of constructivism somewhat resembles the first, although the construction of meaning predominant in the second also has an important role to play. It differs from the first in that the contingent nature of technological change is stressed. The notion in the 'social shaping' approach that technologies physically embody political or other values can be as reductionist as technological determinism. The causality is simply reversed. Instead of technological change causing social effects, the dominant social values result in some sorts of technologies being developed rather than others. The third form of constructivism differs from the second in that the process of stabilising meaning, itself always dynamic and contingent, is central to the process of creating the artefact and does not only occur after the artefact enters a wider world of consumption and use. This notion of 'interpretative flexibility' has been one of the major contributions of the 'social construction of technology' approach (Pinch and Bijker 1987; Bijker 1995).

There is no single position adopted by all the contributors to this book concerning the relationship between technology and society. All of them argue against technological determinism, although some find such a position more difficult to sustain than others. Indeed, Chris Freeman (1987) has written elsewhere in defence of technological determinism and his chapter in this book retains some attachment to that approach. Most also argue against understanding technology as neutral, although, again, there are times when notions of 'choice' about how we use technology seem to suggest a 'technology as neutral' perspective. In most cases, contributors employ some version of constructivism in their analyses. For example, in pointing to the key interest groups shaping the development of the specific technologies of cable and satellite television in Britain and community television in Canada, both Kathy Walker and Herbert Pimlott adopt 'social shaping' perspectives. In contrast, Flis Henwood, Sarah Plumeridge and Linda Stepulevage's chapter on gender inequality in computing education adopts a constructivist framework more concerned with the complex and often contradictory process by which differences and technological inequalities are constructed in discourse and practice, rather than being reflected or embodied in particular technological artefacts and knowledges. We now turn to explore the ways in which technology and in/equality have been analysed in the information society literature.

QUESTIONING THE INFORMATION SOCIETY

At the beginning of this chapter, we provided an account of the British Prime Minister, Tony Blair, taking his first steps into the 'information society', during which he marvelled at the pace and pervasiveness of change brought about by ICTs. Like many of his colleagues in politics and government, he adopts a technologically determinist point of view, granting enormous transformative power to these technologies. In addition, he is keen to promote the notion of an 'information society', regarding it as central to the success of the British economy and the well-being of its citizens. In this chapter, we have already provided a critique of technological determinism and demonstrated the complexity associated with the concept of 'in/equality'. In this section, we turn briefly to the third area of debate central to this volume, namely that of 'information society' itself.

Contradictory claims are made for the 'information society'. On the one hand, the emancipatory potential of the greater availability of ICTs and information is celebrated; on the other hand, warnings are made about the threat to individual liberty and social cohesion. These debates are not new. Their origins can be found in the work of Daniel Bell (1973), who was concerned with the decline of manufacturing activity and employment in the US, the rise of service employment and the centrality of information processing activities to the economy. In his view, the emergence of a 'post-industrial' or 'information' society would be a positive development, accompanied by more social planning and a subordination of capitalist interests to those of meritocracy and welfare. As the industrial society succeeded in meeting people's material needs, so the information society would fulfil people's needs for education, entertainment and personal development.

Subsequent critiques of the empirical basis of Bell's analysis have attacked his undifferentiated approach to services and his focus on the US (for example, in Gershuny and Miles 1983; Lyon 1988; Webster 1995; Poynter and de Miranda in this volume). Neverthe-less, the basic thrust of his argument about the importance of information processing activities in economic, social and political life has endured. Indeed, many of Bell's original predictions about the emerging policy issues remain pertinent. He was concerned about competition, privacy, massification of entertainment, the role of cities and of nation-states. It could be argued that Manuel

Castells (1996) now occupies Bell's position of prophet of social and economic transformation. Castells, however, is more careful to differentiate between different types of information society. Despite common elements, Sweden, the US and Japan each represent very different types of social organisations. Similarly, the nature of what Castells calls 'informational societies' is temporally and spatially contingent.

Although Castells can be accused of technological determinism and does, in fact claim, '[a] technological revolution, centered around information technologies, is reshaping, at accelerated pace, the material basis of society' (Castells 1996: 1), he is not always optimistic and addresses questions of equality and inequality directly. Indeed, in his *Informational City* (1989), he argues that we are seeing the emergence of new class relationships, with a new polarisation of jobs and skills occurring as part of these informational developments. It is, he argues, only the information professionals and managers who control and operate the 'flows of information' who are the 'truly indispensable components of the system' (Castells 1989: 30). Other workers, in the back office as well as in personal service occupations, are perceived as more disposable.

Castells' approach to inequalities in 'informational societies' tends to emphasise social structure, although, in the second volume of his later trilogy (Castells 1997), he is also concerned with questions of self and identity in an increasingly networked world. This is congruent with more recent work, conducted largely within a postmodernist framework, which emphasises the power of technology to create new meanings, new entities and new worlds. One of the most influential authors in this vein is Donna Haraway (1985; 1997) who enthusiastically embraces the indeterminacy and unpredictability of modern technoscience and delights in being a 'cyborg', a hybrid of organism and machine. Sherry Turkle is also enthusiastic about the potential for people 'to express multiple and often unexplored aspects of the self, to play with their identity and to try out new ones' (1995: 12). Such arguments are seductive in their ability to direct our thinking towards new possibilities, but they often ignore the mundane, material reality of many people's lives in which people do not have the personal, cultural or financial resources to engage in such playful activities.

There are, however, critiques of 'information society' that address questions of equality and inequality in ways that combine structural analysis with an analysis of individual and collective agency. A recent collection edited by Brian Loader (1998) is a case in point. Loader and the contributors to that collection take a critical stance in relation to 'the apolitical attitude towards technological development' found in most information society literature (Loader 1998: 6) and questions are raised about access to information and information networks for a range of different groups who are potentially vulnerable in the new 'cyberspace divide'. Attention is drawn to the material disadvantages experienced by the world's 'information poor' (Holderness 1998; Haywood 1998) as well as to the question of women's limited participation in the information society (Adam and Green 1998). However, they argue for more than greater access to, and 'inclusion' in, these developments. Thus, whilst the negative implications of exclusion are examined in a range of contexts, the overall argument of the collection is that 'inclusion' must be a process which is the result of the 'human agency' of the many diverse individuals and cultural or national groups who should help shape and determine, and not merely 'access', technological outcomes. Thus, Loader has predicted, '[t]he development of the information society is not likely to be characterised by a linear technological progression, but rather through the often competing forces of innovation, competitive advantage, human agency and social resistance' (Loader 1998: 15).

In this book, contributors have developed their critiques of information society along similar lines to those found in Loader. Differential access to, and control over, information and ICTs is the focus of most chapters but no simple causal relationship to inequality is assumed. Instead, the various contributors seek to ask if, where and how these particular differences constitute inequalities and, in some cases, offer suggestions as to what might be done to prevent such outcomes. In this context, both individual and collective actions are considered alongside the role of governments, corporations and educational institutions.

THE ORGANISATION OF THE BOOK

This book is divided into three parts, following this introductory chapter. Part I, 'Promises and threats: access and control in media technologies', contains four chapters. First, Graham Thomas and Sally Wyatt challenge common perceptions about the rate of growth of the Internet and about the meaning of 'access' to it, demonstrating that there continue to exist wide differences between the access enjoyed by different social groups. They question the assumptions on which diffusion of Internet connection is seen as necessarily expanding and beneficial. They argue that access is not the only important issue for understanding inequality and illustrate how use of the Internet is affected by the control and ownership of key aspects of its provision.

Rod Allen and Nod Miller look at some of the claims made when information and communications technologies such as radio and cable television were introduced in Britain and North America. They focus particularly on optimistic predictions about the contribution to be made by cable television to the strengthening of local democracy and the extension of the public sphere, and examine the extent to which such promises have been made good. They analyse some of the claims made for the newer Internet technologies and suggest that they have characteristics which create some opportunities for enhancement of democracy and of access to means of distribution of information and ideas.

Kathy Walker explores the tension between an ethos of public service broadcasting which aimed to provide equality of access to high quality diverse programming with the objective of raising cultural standards across the nation, and a market-driven ethos which aims to maximise consumer choice. In the latter, income inequalities play an increasing role in the distribution of access. This shift from a commitment to the general public good to a notion of equality based on individual rights has been accompanied by developments in cable, satellite and digital technologies. The source of these technical changes is not discussed, but what is described is the response of various actors, including the BBC and government committees.

Herbert Pimlott examines the relationship between technology and inequality by investigating the attempts of the community access television movement during the 1960s to 1980s in Canada and the US to redress the communication imbalance between citizens and government. Pimlott draws attention to the special nature of information inequalities, emphasising that it is not simply a question of having access to information. People also need the skills and knowledge to manipulate information for their own purposes. This chapter and the one by Allen and Miller challenge the technologically determinist rhetoric promising greater participation in the public sphere.

Part II, 'Exclusion, inclusion and segregation: new technology and skill in education', focuses on education in ICT skills and the use of ICTs in delivering education. Flis Henwood, Sarah Plumeridge and Linda Stepulevage examine two higher education information technology courses – one traditional computer science course and one interdisciplinary course – in order to explore the relationship between technology and gender inequality. Through an analysis of the notion of 'equal opportunities', the authors demonstrate how technology, technical skill and gender relations are socially constructed. They argue that liberal equal opportunities policies, which aim to increase the numbers of women undertaking IT training, are likely to fail because the cultural nature of both gender and technology are not recognised.

Nod Miller, Helen Kennedy and Linda Leung draw insights from a project which was designed to enhance access to university courses in technology for mature black women in an economically disadvantaged urban area. The project involved the development of distance learning materials delivered to students through computers loaned to them at home. The authors contrast the rhetoric of recent policy documents which suggest that educational inequalities may be easily addressed through the application of ICTs in education with the experience of the complex economic, technical and pedagogic challenges faced by learners and tutors in the course of the project.

In Part III, 'Technology, inequality and economic development', the focus shifts to economic and employment issues. First Chris Freeman extends his previous analysis of long cycles in the economy, in which there is a counter-cyclical relationship between economic growth and technological innovation, to incorporate social inequality. He demonstrates how income and employment inequalities are exacerbated during the diffusion of major new technologies, such as ICTs. Much of his analysis focuses on the UK; however, he also draws attention to the ways in which inequalities between nation-states are manifested through the uneven development of the world economy.

Gavin Poynter and Alvaro de Miranda challenge the view that the application of new technologies in the workplace leads to the end of repetitive jobs and the emancipation of the workforce. They provide a critique of traditional analyses of the division of labour and work processes in the context of the introduction of new ICTs. Their case study of the development of one of the key sites of employment growth – call centres – illustrates the way in which traditional patterns of inequality (for example, between men and women at work) continue and are often reinforced.

In the final chapter, Peter Senker addresses questions about the persistence of poverty and the failure of science and technology policy to be directed towards its alleviation. The development and application of new technologies does lead to economic growth and the resultant benefits do 'trickle down' to some extent to enhance the lives of those in economically disadvantaged groups. But, drawing on examples from agriculture and pharmaceuticals as well as ICTs, he contends that allowing market forces to determine the direction of scientific and technological change leads to the development of processes and products which satisfy the demands of affluent people while threatening the livelihoods of poor people in developing countries.

NOTES

1 Most of this section is adapted from Wyatt (1998: 9–16).
2 In addition, some philosophers have suggested that societies are transformed by technologies, but generally for the worse as technological rationality comes to dominate all spheres of life (Ellul 1964; Mumford 1967).

Part I

PROMISES AND THREATS

Access and control in media technologies

2

ACCESS IS NOT THE ONLY PROBLEM

Using and controlling the Internet

Graham Thomas and Sally Wyatt[1]

We all agreed, as a basic hypothesis, that the Internet should connect all the computers in the world. There are about 200 million of them today, but the number is growing rapidly. Vast portions of the planet are getting richer and more industrialised. There are reasons to believe that at some point in the near future, all Indian schoolboys and all Chinese schoolgirls will use their own laptop computers at school. In fact, when we plan the new Internet, it would be immoral not to consider that all humans will eventually be connected ...

A figure of a hundred computers per human is not entirely unreasonable, leading to a thousand billion computers in the Internet in 2020. But some have observed that such a target was a bit narrow, that we wanted safety margins. Eventually, the official objectives for IPng (Internet Protocol, new generation) were set to one quadrillion computers (10 to the power 15) connected through one trillion networks (10 to the power 12).

(Huitema 1998: 2–3)

The designers of the Internet of the future, as they debated the key parameters of the new Internet protocol IPng (now usually known as IPv6, Internet Protocol version 6), revealed both technical caution and their inclusive aspirations for the Internet. The language in the above quotation transcends typical technical discourse and explicitly brings in social and ethical considerations: 'it would be *immoral* not to consider that all humans will eventually be connected'. The IPv6 designers certainly wanted to ensure that Internet address space, if nothing else, would not become a scarce resource in the foreseeable future.

The aspirations of the Internet's designers perhaps go even further. In a series of speeches during 1998, the co-designer of the original Internet protocol, Vinton Cerf, announced the start of work designed to take the Internet beyond the Earth's boundaries. (Details of progress towards this goal at NASA's Jet Propulsion Laboratory and the technical problems which would need to be solved are provided by Iannotta 1999.) Whether the facilities of the proposed 'InterPlaNet' will be accessed by extra-terrestrial civilisations is a question which will not be addressed in this chapter. Nonetheless, the intention to expand and to include as many users as possible is clearly evident.

Furthermore, as part of a restructuring of the closest thing the Internet has to a governing body, the Internet Society, an Internet Societal Task Force was created in 1999 to complement the existing engineering and research task forces. One of its aims was to address problems confronting the realisation of the Internet Society's new slogan: 'The Internet is for Everyone' (Cerf 1999).

Such inclusive intentions have often been voiced during the evolution of the Internet since the 1960s. The original ARPANET may have had its origins in the field of military communications during the Cold War, but it was quickly converted into a network, and then a set of networks, covering a much wider constituency. Despite the key contribution of the US government as a central actor, the spread of the Internet was a very decentralised and open process. A new network could 'join' the Internet if its owners could find a site already on the Internet which was willing to exchange traffic and if they installed the publicly available Internet software protocols. The rapid growth of the Internet and its commercialisation in the 1990s have changed somewhat the basis on which Internet traffic is exchanged, but so far the accessibility of the Internet to new entrants has not been essentially compromised.

The apparently endless expansion of the Internet is not the whole story. A wealth of statistics point to the gap between the noble aspirations expressed by Huitema and Cerf and the unequal distribution of access to the Internet within and between individual societies. This chapter aims to gauge the extent and severity of the problem of unequal access but also to go beyond the 'access problem' to point out actual and potential inequalities inherent in the current structure of the Internet and its services, and the ways in which inequalities might be exacerbated or reduced as the Internet is shaped over the coming years. We stress the connectedness of the Internet in its entirety, through an exploration of the relationship between inequalities in the use of the Internet and those associated with its production. Access to and ownership of telephones, television, home computers and Internet accounts are all seen as indicators of inequality within and between social groups. We suggest that inequalities in consumption patterns are not only a function of, *inter alia*, place, education, race, income and gender, but are also bound up with the structures of the production of the Internet itself. Before exploring these issues, we outline a history of the Internet, focusing on shifting patterns of consumption and production.

A BRIEF HISTORY OF INTERNET TIME[2]

The explosive growth of the Internet since the mid-1990s can be bewildering for users, producers and commentators. The services available, the tools needed to build it and gain access to it, and the composition of the Internet industry are all mutating very rapidly. Some commentators speak in terms of 'Internet years' – units of time much shorter than calendar years but which nonetheless contain enough changes to fill a year in most other industries. One of the consequences of this explosive growth is that at any moment during the past decade a large proportion of Internet users was new to it. Anyone who uses it for more than a few months will find the need to learn how to use new software. The changes are probably even greater for those who provide Internet-based services, who have to adjust to the proliferation of new languages, protocols and standards.

The vast majority of present Internet users and producers experience it as something new and dynamic. Yet the Internet has a long history and some parts of it are extremely stable. Precisely when the Internet began is open to interpretation, but the latest plausible date is early 1982, when the Internet protocols still used today were formally introduced. Earlier start dates might include 1972, when the first connection between ARPANET and another network (ALOHAnet in Hawaii) was opened, or 1969 when the first four nodes of ARPANET were connected to one another.

Whichever date is chosen, the point is that the Internet is not a completely new phenomenon.[3]

Dempsey (1993) identifies four main stages of Internet development.[4] In modified form, and with our own approximate dates, these are:

1. the Internet as testbed or *scientists' playground* where the technical problems of creating a wide area computer network were being solved (most of the 1970s, primarily in the US);
2. the emergence of an Internet *community*, consisting mostly of computing science professionals and students, when new services and new forms of communications such as Usenet groups began to develop (from the end of the 1970s to around 1987, concentration in the US remained but increasingly other industrialised countries became involved);
3. the broadening of the Internet into a *general academic resource*, when the information and services on the Internet became more important than the addresses of the connected computers (from about 1987 to 1993, predominantly in industrialised countries);
4. the transformation of the Internet into a *commercial information infrastructure* (since the availability of the World Wide Web in 1993, theoretically worldwide but in practice still highly concentrated in industrialised countries).

The decision of the US National Science Foundation in 1991 to allow commercial traffic heralded the switch of the Internet from an academically-oriented network to a commercially-oriented one. This was followed by the creation of the Commercial Internet Exchange to regulate the exchange of traffic between the newly emerging commercial Internet service providers (ISPs) and to act as an ISP association. The number of service providers grew very rapidly, and they began to differentiate the market according to whether they operated nationally or regionally and whether they provided services to individuals or organisations. These US developments were followed, sooner or later, in other countries.

The explosive growth in the commercial Internet came after the World Wide Web (one of the last innovations from the 'academic' era) became accessible via a graphical user interface in 1993. The combination of this interface and the extensibility of the Web which allowed it to incorporate multimedia features and to integrate previously separate services such as information access, file transfer and electronic mail, meant that it became easy to demonstrate the potential of the Internet to prospective users. Firms quickly saw the advantages of having an 'online brochure' which could advertise their goods and services around the world at low cost. Finding ways of making real money on or via the Internet (aside from speculative stock market valuations) has proved more difficult for most commercial users, although much effort is being devoted to this goal.

By any of the common measures – such as the number of connected computers, separate networks or users – the Internet has grown dramatically. Four computers were connected to one another at the end of 1969; the number grew to 188 by 1979, 159,000 by 1989 and over fifty-six million by mid-1999 (Zakon 1999). This growth has not been evenly distributed. Of all the Internet hosts (computers with Internet addresses) using generic domain names, 79 per cent were identifiably in the commercial sector (.com or .net) in July 1999, up from 47 per cent in January 1995. The public sector share (.edu, .mil, .gov and .int) fell from 48 per cent in 1995 to 17 per cent in 1999. Non-profit-making organisations accounted for around 5 per cent in 1995 and only 2 per cent in 1999. Despite the limitations of the data,[5] they do provide an indication of the growth of the commercial sector from a very low base at the end of the 1980s to a position of dominance less than ten years later.

A vociferous debate has been taking place within sections of the Internet-using population about the effects of commercialisation on the traditions and practices which made the Internet successful in the first place. Some attribute the Internet's rapid growth to lack of government control and the free competition of both ideas and products in the marketplace. Others stress the importance of the public-sector history of the Internet, including government finance and the openness of non-proprietary Internet protocols and standards. From a commercial perspective, the 'old' Internet has been described as 'not ready for business' because it was too open, too amateur and too steeped in academic/nerd culture. In contrast, others worry that commercial pressures will lead to an Internet which is mean-spirited and which will exacerbate inequalities and disenfranchise groups within society (Barbrook 1996; Borsook 1996; Hudson 1997). We cannot assume that the dramatic increase in the number of host computers is evenly distributed within and between social groups. In the next section, we examine the available data to see who does have access to the Internet. Later, we focus on the groups involved in the production of the Internet, especially service and content providers. We also explore the forces pulling the Internet in different directions, such as electronic commerce and new infrastructure possibilities, in order to assess the extent to which the Internet can remain open for users with divergent aims and with unequal access to ownership and control of such resources.

CONSUMING THE INTERNET

The dramatic increase in the number of Internet hosts in recent years tempts many commentators to conclude that this rate of growth will continue, or even accelerate. As the quotation at the beginning of the chapter suggests, the designers of the Internet are indeed planning for continued growth. It is assumed the Internet is following a very common path, one followed by many other successful technologies before it. Economists refer to this path as 'trickle down'[6]: the process whereby technologies which are initially expensive to use become cheaper over time, simultaneously providing more people with the benefits of the technology and enlarging the market.[7] In the case of the Internet, the early users were a small number of academics who used computers paid for largely from university budgets or defence contracts. Now, users include all sorts of academics as well as firms, political and voluntary groups and individuals at home.

According to the trickle-down view, there may be inequalities of access and use during the early stages of a technology but it is assumed these disappear, or are at least much reduced, as the technology becomes more widely diffused. Internet enthusiasts often claim that connection is a global process, albeit an uneven one. This is not unique to the Internet. Similar claims can be found in much literature and in policy statements about industrialisation and modernisation more generally. Individuals, regions and nations will 'catch up'; those who are not connected now will, or should be, soon. This is the real annihilation of space by time: the assumption that the entire world shares a single timeline of development, in which some groups are further ahead than others along this shared path.

John Perry Barlow, co-founder of the Electronic Frontier Foundation, is committed to the emancipatory potential of the Internet. But he, too, adopts the trickle-down perspective and downplays the transient inconveniences some people will experience. 'Will there be data sweatshops? Probably. But, just as the sweatshops of New York were a way station for families whose progeny are now on Long Island, so, too, will these pass' (1998: 158).

These views of trickling-down or catching-up contain three fallacies. The first is that growth is evenly distributed, whereas most of the available data suggest that it is not. Evidence for the catching-up assumption is furnished – at least within the so-called advanced industrial societies – by time series of statistics relating to ownership of consumer goods such as motor vehicles, televisions and refrigerators, all of which were once owned by very small percentages of households but are now much more widely diffused. Globally, however, the catching up effect would seem to be less obvious, and measurement of ownership of consumer goods *per se* says nothing about inequalities in the type and quality of goods possessed. What is the situation with regard to the Internet? A word of caution about what follows: collecting and interpreting data about Internet use is not straightforward. Defining a host, ascertaining its location, identifying users and their demographic characteristics are all fraught with difficulty. Nonetheless, some patterns can be discerned.

Differences between countries remain stark. The 1999 report from the United Nations Development Program (UNDP) illustrates this: in mid-1998, industrialised countries – with less than 15 per cent of the world's population – accounted for 88 per cent of Internet users. The US, with less than 5 per cent of the world's people, had more than a quarter of the world's Internet users. South Asia, on the other hand, had more than 20 per cent of the world's population but less than 1 per cent of its Internet users. (UNDP 1999: 62–3) Big differences exist even between OECD countries: in the US and Nordic countries, more than a quarter of the population had Internet access whereas in the UK it was given as only 10 per cent (UNDP 1999: 63).

Gender differences have shown the most dramatic reduction. Georgia Technical University (1999) has been conducting online surveys of Internet users approximately every six months since January 1994. In the first survey, only 5 per cent of users were women. In October 1998, women represented just over one third of users worldwide (33.6 per cent). Nonetheless, the stereotypical user remains a young, white, university-educated man. Even though more and more women are using the Internet, women may still be struggling with the feeling that they do not really belong there; and this may be particularly the case outside of the US and Canada. Since the sixth survey, conducted in October 1996, gender differences have been broken down according to region. In Europe, less than 20 per cent of users were women in 1996; and this proportion was much the same, 18.4 per cent, in October 1998. (The figures should again be treated with caution; European sample sizes are very small, as the vast majority of respondents to the GTU surveys comes from the US and Canada).

Differences based on race and income remain very marked. The first national survey in the US to collect data on ethnicity and Internet use was conducted during December 1996/January 1997, based on nearly 6000 respondents. Hoffman and Novak (1998) analyse this data and conclude that race continues to matter. Whites are more likely to own home computers and to have used the Internet than African Americans, even allowing for differences in education. The most worrying result occurs amongst high school and college students who do not have access to a home computer. Nearly 38 per cent of white students, compared with only 16 per cent of African American students, find some alternative means of accessing the Internet. This may reflect different patterns of access within schools, or – the explanation favoured by Hoffman and Novak – different schools may have variable levels of Internet-related resources.

A similar picture emerged from larger surveys (of approximately 48,000 households) conducted by the US Census Bureau on behalf of the National Telecommunications and Information Administration (NTIA) in 1994, 1997 and 1998. The analysis of these surveys highlights what the authors call a 'persisting digital divide'. They note substantial increases in PC and modem ownership and e-mail access, but go on to state:

> Despite this significant growth in computer ownership and usage overall, the growth has occurred to a greater extent within some income levels, demographic groups and geographic areas, than in others. In fact, the 'digital divide' between certain groups of Americans has *increased* between 1994 and 1997 so that there is now an even greater disparity in penetration levels among some groups.
>
> (NTIA 1998: summary)

NTIA has found that there is still a significant 'digital divide' separating American information 'haves' and 'have nots.' Indeed, in many instances, the digital divide has widened in the last year.

(NTIA 1999a: summary)

The second fallacy implicit in the trickle-down assumption about continued growth is precisely that growth will indeed continue. In 1998, *Which? Online* (Consumers' Association 1998) suggested that 14 per cent of the UK population have access to the Internet at home or at work. In line with other market analysts, it predicts that this will double within two years. But why should that be the case? (Consumers' Association 1998). The *Which? Online* survey also found that 25 per cent of non-users did not realise a computer was necessary to gain access and 63 per cent of non-users did not realise a telephone line was required. Nearly a quarter of all respondents feared that use of the Internet would lead to antisocial behaviour. Popular wisdom suggests that access is the problem: overcoming people's fear and ignorance, making the technology cheaper and easier to use, will all contribute to continuing growth in the numbers of users. The assumption that once people have access and have learned to use the technology, its value will be self-evident and they will embrace it enthusiastically may not be the case. Maybe the usefulness and pleasure of the Internet is not for everyone. Some technologies experience an early bout of enthusiastic uptake but then fade away, including CB radio, community video (see Pimlott, this volume) and videotex.

Nearly all the academic and policy literature focuses on how to increase the number of users, assuming that once a user, always a user. For example, the conclusions of Hoffman and Novak are to 'ensure access and use will follow' (1998: 9). Moreover, they conclude, 'programs that encourage home computer ownership ... and the adoption of inexpensive devices that enable Internet access over the television should be aggressively pursued, especially for African Americans' (1998: 9). Other empirical work suggests that providing access may not be the sure, simple solution it appears. Based on two national, random telephone surveys, Katz and Aspden (1998) suggest there are patterns to non-use. People who stop using the Internet are poorer and less well-educated. People who are introduced to the Internet via family and friends are more likely to drop out than those who are self-taught or who receive formal training at work or school. Teenagers are more likely to give up than people over twenty. The reasons people abandon the Internet are, in descending order of importance, that they lose institutional access, they find it boring or difficult to use or it is too expensive. Many ex-users have computers at home which they continue to use for other purposes, but not for Internet access.[8] These data need to be treated with caution – former users can of course become active users again at a later date – but they are interesting because they call into question the assumption of never-ending growth. They also suggest that public access provision, quality of information and training remain important policy issues. If the results about teenagers are replicated elsewhere on a large scale, certain assumptions about the rate of exponential growth have to be re-examined. Maybe the Internet is one of many things with which teenagers experiment only to abandon or use in moderation as they become older.

The third fallacy implicit in the trickle-down approach is that the absolute increase in numbers of Internet users will necessarily lead to less inequality. In general, the creation of conditions for 'unfettered' growth might initially exacerbate inequalities, and, even after this initial stage, trickle-down actually implies the continuance of inequalities across the full spectrum of desirable products: by the time an old product has trickled down to the lower layers, a newer one has been innovated and, by its scarcity, has become an indicator of high status. Furthermore, espousal of the trickle-down approach has policy consequences, most obviously a wait-and-see attitude to the alleviation of inequality. If access to a previously scarce resource is increasing year on year, is it not better to wait and see at what level the rate of increase starts to slow down and only then take action to bridge the gap between the 'natural' level of access provided by the market and the level deemed socially desirable? This argument has been made in relation to universal service obligations for advanced tele-communications services (Noam 1994).

With regard to the Internet, there is a more fundamental issue related to its changing nature as it has moved away from universities and into its commercial world. During the 1970s and 1980s, the Internet was used by a small, privileged group: academics used it to share computer resources and to share data. It was one of a number of academic tools but not one which fundamentally altered existing power relations. As the Internet has become more widely used during the 1990s and is promoted as the ideal medium for information and commerce by many politicians, lack of access may contribute, in both actuality and perception, to exclusion from sources of information, debate and access to goods and services, particularly if Internet delivery becomes a substitute for more traditional supply channels. This is one reason why it is important to examine how access to resources necessary for shaping the future direction of the Internet are distributed and manipulated by the major actors involved.

Before moving on to this, let us examine how one key determinant of the extent of inequality in Internet access – cost – might develop. The costs of gaining access to the Internet can be broken down into the following components: equipment charges, software charges, telecommunications charges and charges levied by Internet access providers.

The cost of equipment was one of the main reasons why organisations gained access to the Internet before individual consumers. It is only fairly recently, and only in the richest countries, that ownership of personal computers has become relatively common. Even now, only a few countries have ownership levels approaching 50 per cent of households; in Britain only 27 per cent of households owned a PC in 1999 (McIntosh 1999). Only since 1997 has the cost of modems fallen to the level where they are routinely included in 'consumer' PCs. The next wave of access is predicted to come on the back of the diffusion of digital television, but this diffusion itself is subject to public acceptance, and the fall in costs to a level where most consumers can afford it is (at the time of writing) still some years away. However, diffusion of Internet-capable computers is continuing, helped by pressures to provide children with what are seen as essential facilities for their education. Software for Internet access is generally perceived as 'free', i.e. it is bundled with new computers and/or provided as part of Internet access packages.

Telecommunications costs are (in most of the world) a disincentive for residential users and small organisations. Large organisations generally obtain fixed-cost leased-line access in order to gain enough capacity for their members and to control their budgets. Individuals and small organisations, at least for the immediate future, have to use standard telephone lines which, in most countries (with the USA and Canada being the chief exceptions) means paying for metered calls. Telephone charging systems were created for a market mainly comprised of voice calls. The longer average call durations of Internet sessions incur often dramatically higher costs and therefore metered local call charges act as a general disincentive to access; such charges also structure usage patterns differently from countries where local telephony is unmetered. While there is much consumer pressure to reduce or abolish such charges, telephone companies are reluctant to do away with such an abundant source of extra revenue. New telecommunications provision on the basis of 'cable modems' and the xDSL family of protocols is being delivered on an 'always on' basis, which means flat-fee rather than metered access charges, but it remains to be seen if and how fast prices will fall to levels which make such access generally affordable.

Telecommunications costs are also a source of inequality *between* nations because of the way in which individual networks connect to the rest of the Internet. The main Internet exchange points are in the USA, and every major Internet service provider, wherever it is in the world, needs to connect to at least one of these points. Providers based outside the USA must pay for international leased lines, which – although costs are falling due to increased competition and the installation of new capacity – are considerably more expensive than lines inside the USA. (This is actually a less equitable arrangement than used to be the case in the 1980s when the US National Science Foundation shared the costs of Internet links to other national research networks.)

The costs of Internet service provision itself have developed in an interesting way. In Britain, the first commercial ISPs were initially more concerned with covering their costs than with making money: Demon Internet estimated that for its hoped-for initial market it would need to charge each user ten pounds per month (plus taxes) to pay for Demon's equipment and its single 64k leased line. This 'tenner a month' fee became the standard charge for the companies that followed; apart from the existing 'online service providers' (such as AOL and Compuserve) which continued to charge hourly fees and extra money for specific content, flat-rate access charges became the norm and remained relatively low (a few 'premium' companies charged as much as fifteen pounds a month plus taxes, but most stayed at or below than Demon's figure).[9]

Even so, access charges, coming as they did on top of time-based telephone charges, restricted the number of people willing to pay for domestic Internet access (they also restricted organisational access in the case of small businesses and voluntary organisations). The extent of this was shown dramatically from mid-1998 when an opportunity, created accidentally by telecommunications legislation concerning the distribution of revenues for calls passed from one telecommunications operator to another, allowed a number of UK organisations to offer 'free' Internet access.[10] The leading 'free' ISP, Dixons Freeserve, announced that it had signed up a million new customers within a few months of starting the service. Even allowing for churn, second accounts and displacement from other ISPs, this was impressive evidence of both a high level of demand and the barriers to access presented even by low charges. Users of 'free' ISPs still have to buy equipment and pay telephone costs, but the elimination of subscription charges helps to reduce differences in access costs between Britain and North America. It will be interesting to see if this model is emulated elsewhere (in 1999 a small number of 'free' providers were operating in continental Europe); much depends on the attitudes of national telecommunications regulators. In the meantime, the number of 'free' ISPs in Britain was increasing throughout 1999, with large companies from other sectors (supermarkets, newspapers, banks, football clubs, etc.) taking the opportunity to provide 'own brand' Internet access for their customers, in collaboration with a much smaller number of companies providing technical services and call termination.

In the longer term, the 'flat rate' Internet access model may be put at risk by developments in the way Internet service providers connect to each other. Put simply, unlike national telephone companies, Internet service providers do not charge each other for terminating traffic originated by other providers. This is largely because the Internet developed in the context of public funding, and the non-commercial owners of the various interconnecting networks viewed billing for traffic as a deterrent to use and an unnecessary administrative burden rather than as a source of revenue. There is potential for unfairness here, with smaller networks effectively getting a 'free ride' by giving their customers access to resources hosted within larger and/or more popular networks. In the new commercial context of today's Internet, this poses a problem for ISPs and telcos who want to maximise their own revenue. At present, the resentment of the larger networks has not resulted in the introduction of telephony-style 'settlements'. Instead, these networks have created interconnect 'clubs' with relatively high barriers to entry; this gives them more efficient connections to other parts of the Internet and encourages smaller networks to become their subsidiaries. In future, settlements might be introduced, which would have implications for both the basis and level of access (or usage) charges. The entry of mainstream telecommunications companies into the fledgling 'Internet telephony' market may also put pressure on the traditional flat-rate charging model.

The costs of access to the Internet, and their implications for the lessening or exacerbation of inequality of access, are clearly very important but, as the title of this chapter suggests, access is not the only problem. There are other dimensions to inequality in relation to the Internet. The next section looks at issues affecting inequality in the provision and use of Internet services.

PRODUCING THE INTERNET

During the early 1980s, when the Internet was mostly confined within the computer science community, there was relatively little distinction between the producers of Internet services and content and the consumers. If you had the skills and resources necessary to access the Internet, it was more than likely that you would have the skills and resources necessary to produce content and (sometimes) services for it. Academics collaborated to share resources, and much use of the Internet was for interactive personal communication. There was an ethos of 'give some, take some' and of exchange of software and ideas.

This tradition was extended by the appearance of the World Wide Web, which made it easy for almost anyone with a small amount of technical knowledge to become an 'Internet publisher'. The first versions of HTML, the mark-up language of Web documents, may not have contained all the features which desktop publishing experts were used to, but they did make it easy to create documents and to link them to other documents. Document and resource sharing was of course the impetus behind the creation of the Web; the original graphical Web browser, Mosaic, even contained an annotation provision which allowed readers to work actively (offline) with documents they had accessed.

Since then, things have changed somewhat. Many Web authors demanded more features and greater control over the appearance of their documents, and both programmers and users wished to be able to make their pages more interactive and more flexibly tailored to users' requirements. The increased emphasis on scripting languages, multimedia and links between the Web interface and organisational databases (enabling the automated creation of customised Web pages 'on the fly') has meant that skilled programmers have more than regained any ground they may have lost to the mass of user-producers in the Web's early days. It is not that simple documents cannot now be published. The development of graphically-based Web authoring programs means that simple pages can be produced with even less technical knowledge than before. There is a growing differentiation, however, between such basic Web production and the more sophisticated production which is seen as the basis for competitive advantage for commercial firms and other organisations competing for attention, time and custom.

It was perhaps inevitable that the expansion of the Internet would lead to an increased division between producers and consumers of Internet services – especially once growth of usage reached the stage where new users were learning to use the Internet at the same time as they were learning to use computers. In Britain, anecdotal evidence suggests there may be a correlation between the rise of 'free' services and the notion of the Internet as essentially a site of consumption. In an article comparing 'free' with paid-for Internet access, the author notes, 'Mailing lists tend to be full of people posting from business accounts and paid-for ISPs rather than free ones, which might reflect the kind of users free services attract – takers rather than contributors' (Patient 1999: 35).

The enthusiasm of the early days of the Web, when it was commonly thought that this new medium would reduce the power of the largest organisations and provide an opportunity for smaller organisations and individuals to create and prosper on a 'level playing field', now needs to be tempered by the existence of an increasing gap between producers and consumers; in particular, the fact that the creation of a state-of-the-art Web site may require considerable resources returns the advantage to organisations with deep pockets and widens the 'opportunity gap'.

This trend is reinforced by other trends in the area of resource provision. In earlier times, Internet content most definitely had to be (inter)actively 'pulled' by the user rather than being 'pushed' at the user by the provider. Documents and other resources had to be fetched by the user (who had to know not only the name of the underlying file but also its exact location). Obviously, information about the location of resources had to be spread somehow – first via messages in newsgroups and on bulletin boards, later by the first indexing programs such as *archie*.

With the explosion in the amount of 'content' made possible by the Web, new means had to be found to allow users to find what they were looking for. The Web's hypertext links were of course themselves useful in this regard, but 'surfing' from one page to another in search of useful resources was an inefficient method. Two approaches were adopted by the creators of the new 'search engines'. The first, exemplified by *Yahoo!*, was to extend the hierarchical indexing method pioneered by software such as *gopher*: resources were collected first into large categories, then broken down into more and more detailed classifications, effectively creating a catalogue. The second, exemplified by AltaVista, was to index documents and then provide a facility for users to enter search terms and to narrow down their queries by more detailed specifications.

The latter approach is more powerful, but it does require a certain amount of skill on the part of the user. The attraction of the catalogue approach for new users is clear. The catalogues provide an obvious answer to the question asked by most new users: 'where do I start?' Both sorts of search engines have proved popular, and some convergence has taken place as Yahoo! now also has a search facility and AltaVista a catalogue. It is an extension of the catalogue approach which is behind one of the main trends in the provision of Web content at the time of writing – the creation of so-called 'portals'. The idea is to provide a comprehensive set of resources accessible from a single site (though not necessarily located at that site). If users can be persuaded to visit a particular portal as their first stop on the Internet (ideally, if they have that site installed as their default 'home page'), then the owners of that portal can maximise revenue from display and 'click-through' advertising and from their role as intermediaries in electronic commerce applications. There is an affinity between access provision and portal provision: default home pages are built into the software installed by access providers, and all the large-scale access providers have been trying to establish themselves also as portals. Of course, it is possible to change the default home page in the browser, but unlike in earlier times a substantial percentage of new users is unable or unwilling to tinker with the provided package of software and settings. A survey in 1999 found that 83% of 874 current UK Web users had not changed their default home page since installing the browser provided by their ISP (NOP 1999).

The result of the scramble for portal supremacy has been a concentration of resources, with mergers and takeovers being announced at a rapid rate. The leading contenders, including AOL, Yahoo! and Microsoft, have been acquiring (with the money provided by high – perhaps over-inflated – stock market valuations) other firms with the aim of putting together a panoply of search facilities, multimedia content, software and access provision. They are being joined in this endeavour by other search engines and by a number of media-related companies including the Disney-ABC network. The linkages between access provision and content provision are being reinforced by the rise of digital television and the promise of the convergence of broadcast and interactive services.

The portal model, and the heavy presence of traditional media organisations, gives impetus to the idea of 'pushing' content – including advertising – at customers rather than waiting for them to pull it down. Once they become used to the idea of going to the portal before going anywhere else they become in effect a captive audience. It has been tried before. So-called 'push technology' was one of the buzzwords of 1996–7: it referred to the creation of 'channels' of Internet content which could be pre-chosen then automatically downloaded without further user intervention. The concept initially foundered because of scarcity of Internet bandwidth, inadequate computer power at the client end and the reluctance of users in countries with metered telephone charges to leave their computers online. But it may be making a return under the umbrella of portals, digital television and 'always on' xDSL and cable modem access.

The process of concentration clearly exacerbates the inequality between large and small content providers. What effect it will have on the availability and cost of resources used by different kinds of customers remains to be seen. So far, the growth of the Internet has led to a huge increase in the amount of resources available to users at low marginal cost. To many people's surprise, the extension of the Internet beyond academia and into the commercial world seemed to slow down, at least temporarily, the steady increase in the commodification of information that had been a feature of advanced 'service economies'. Existing providers of often expensive business-to-business information via dedicated networks or proprietary access modes were forced to rethink their strategies in the wake of the explosion of information carried over the Web. Customers old and new demanded access via the Web, where information suppliers faced a different environment. There was an enormous amount of competition provided by numerous content suppliers using standard software and protocols, and it was difficult to charge for content provision (as opposed to access provision) on the Internet. Pay sites initially had to rely on 'lumpy' investment decisions by users (for example, subscription services) and on the use of payment systems involving credit cards which, rightly or wrongly, provoked fears about security and fraud. Also, it proved difficult for all but the largest organisations to defend intellectual copyright on Internet content.

However, these initial trends are not irreversible. Much effort has been put into the provision of more sophisticated electronic commerce facilities. Already, encryption schemes and secure payment systems have alleviated some fears about the transmission of credit card details over the Internet: fast-growing firms like the Amazon online bookstore have shown that, with secure servers and encryption built into browser software in standard formats, credit card fraud need not be a major problem. Even though e-commerce is already growing quite rapidly, the key breakthrough will occur when it becomes technically and economically efficient to charge small amounts online for small(ish) pieces of information and other Internet content. The problems should not be underestimated; software would need to be standardised, the security question would have to be convincingly addressed, means of accurately assigning ownership of intellectual property would need to be developed and standardised, the co-operation of financial organisations would need to be secured, and the disinclination of consumers to make constant buying decisions during an online session would have to be taken into account. But the rewards are so great (for content providers, portal owners and especially for the firms whose trading systems set the electronic commerce standard) that it is probable that such payment systems will be innovated sooner rather than later.

Concentration of access and portal providers helps to drive this process, because it allows firms which develop successful e-commerce products to dominate larger shares of the market. Once online payment systems are standardised and diffused, the amount of 'paid-for' content will inevitably increase. There may even be a return to the old 'content provider' model where access providers were also repositories of content which only their customers could access. This model was never completely eclipsed by the Internet, surviving in the likes of AOL and Compuserve, but it did for a while become unfashionable. Some of the new 'free' access providers (for example, the service run by the Sun newspaper in the UK) have begun to offer content which is available only to customers using their access facility, presumably to maximise telecommunications revenue, and at least one UK bank is restricting its online banking services to customers using its access gateway. Although the growth of paid-for Internet content may help to cheapen the costs of initial access to the Internet (and perhaps prolong 'free' access beyond the lifetime of current tele-communications regulations), it will also make it possible for inequality of access to specific Internet resources to increase, as some individuals and smaller/poorer organisations will be reluctant to pay the extra money required.

A further development which may work in the same direction goes under the innocuous name of 'quality of service'. This term refers to facilities made technically possible in new versions of the Internet Protocol and underlying transport mechanisms to provide guaranteed end-to-end bandwidth for specific services. The orig-inal aim was to make it possible to provide real-time audio and video services over the Internet, where traditionally such services have been sub-optimal because the delivery time of any individual packet across the Internet could not be guaranteed. The new quality of service provisions will allow the implementation of high-quality real-time services, but they will also allow providers to offer high-speed services of all kinds, probably at premium rates.

Rich organisations have always been able to buy faster Internet connections. But the benefit of such connections extended only as far as the reach of the organisation's own network connections (and maybe those of its direct partners). The speed of any specific packet of data sent across the Internet is only as fast as the slowest segment of the journey, and if data was being sent from a slow site or via a slow intermediate network, then even the fastest network at the user end would not be able to speed its delivery. In that sense, all Internet services hitherto have been 'best-effort' services: nothing could be guaranteed outside the sphere of influence of the user's own network. The distinctive feature of 'quality of service' provisions is the guarantee of *end-to-end* delivery times. The opportunity is there for the bigger networks to collaborate in the offering of high-speed and premium cost services. How much this matters depends on the context: the economy class passenger on a regular transatlantic air service may well arrive at exactly the same destination as the supersonic Concorde passenger – but if time is important, the Concorde passenger may be able to clinch a deal before the economy-class rival touches down.

Finally, in this section dealing with actual and potential inequalities in the way the Internet is produced and shaped, it should not be forgotten that as the Internet has expanded it has become more embedded in existing systems of national and international laws and regulations. The notion of the Internet as an anarchic, self-regulating entity, while remaining persuasive to some people (see Barlow 1996 together with the critique by Barbrook 1996, 1998), is less accurate now than it ever was. The original informal standards-setting procedure of the Internet is not dead, but it is increasingly under strain as Internet standards become increasingly enmeshed with world telecommunications standards and as their development becomes a key element in the strategy of commercial hardware and software providers. Elements of the Internet's structure, such as the administration of domain names, have become important issues for organisations such as the World Trade Organisation and the World Intellectual Property Organisation as well as for national governments. In the extensive debate over the restructuring of the domain name system during 1998 the loudest voices were those of the firms and governments of the advanced industrialised countries. (There is extensive documentation of this debate at the NTIA Web site – NTIA 1999b.) The point here is not that the development of the Internet is necessarily going to be determined by the interests of one or more of the main national and international powers, but that any attempts to create and implement policies for using the Internet to alleviate inequality must take into account the existing interests which will be affected by such policies.

INEQUALITY, HEGEMONY AND FLEXIBILITY

This chapter has attempted to demonstrate how access to and use of the Internet are affected by access to the control and ownership of key aspects of the provision of the Internet. The above sections have perhaps painted a one-sided picture of recent developments in Internet access and service provision. The number and breadth of Internet resources is still growing, and countries around the world are increasing their numbers of Internet users at rates which are faster than those of the United States and other OECD countries, although in some cases the low base of usage means that fast rates of increase do not compensate in terms of absolute numbers. As usage grows outside the North American heartland, the amount of locally-oriented content should also grow commensurately, although this may depend on how far local content producers see

themselves as operating in a global marketplace. But the developments outlined in the earlier sections serve as a corrective to the
over-optimistic view that the Internet will necessarily improve
access to the world's storehouse of knowledge for everyone – rich
or poor, black or white, western or otherwise. It may well be that
some of the factors which made the Internet a success in the first
place – for freely-available information, flat-rate access charges,
co-operation between providers – were the product of the
Internet's public sector origins and will not survive beyond the first
years of the new commercial environment. The UNDP expresses
serious reservations about the inclusive potential of the Internet:

> The typical Internet user worldwide is male, under 35
> years old, with a college education and high income,
> urban-based and English-speaking – a member of a very
> elite minority worldwide. The consequence? The network
> society is creating parallel communications systems: one
> for those with income, education and – literally – connec-
> tions, giving plentiful information at low cost and high
> speed; the other for those without connections, blocked by
> high barriers of time, cost and uncertainty and dependent
> on outdated information.
>
> (UNDP 1999: 63)

Set against this gloomy prediction, though, are factors such as the
weight of history – 'path dependent' structures and traditions
which seem to be relatively tenacious (for example, the absence of
settlements, the continuing influence of the original Internet ethos
of free information exchange) – the cheapening of certain costs
brought about by mass diffusion and economies of scale, and the
growing recognition by politicians, interest groups and regulators
that the Internet matters (in terms of, for example, quality of life
and national competitiveness) and will need regulating if its benefits are to be maximised.

National and international telecommunications regulators are
starting to consider whether Internet access provision should be
written into 'universal service' regulations – although as yet most
have not considered it necessary, believing that it is too soon after
the Internet has attained 'critical mass' (see OFTEL 1999, ch.5).
Other agencies are attempting to ensure that access is provided to
schools, libraries, hospitals, etc., and many towns, cities and
regions have local policies and consortia aimed at boosting access

levels and ensuring that traditional 'have-nots' are not excluded from life online. In our own backyard, for example, the University of East London has close relations with the ambitious Newham Online (1999) initiative, which is attempting to be both a provider of and catalyst for online services in one of the poorer London boroughs.

At the global level, organisations such as the Association of Progressive Communications are pooling the efforts of national non-profitmaking groups to provide support structures and communications systems which aim to provide deprived sections of the world with some level of online access (APC 1999). They point out that much can be achieved with very basic equipment and low-speed telecommunications links: the 'information superhighway' might well be necessary to deliver elaborately-formatted e-mail with pictorial attachments, but the same message content could also be delivered via a slow, store-and-forward, text-only service, courtesy of the 'information dirt-track'. If nothing else, the Internet at least makes it possible for diligent searchers to find information, resources, advice and opinions which challenge the prevailing interpretations of powerful actors. The UNDP report also provides some examples of creative, indirect Internet use, for instance:

> In rural Bolivia, most farmers have never seen a computer, but they already have access to the Internet. How? Farmers with crop concerns can give questions to a community leader, who relays the inquiry to the radio station, where it is sent to UNDP's communications centre. The question is posted on the Internet and answers received are emailed back to the radio station and broadcast.
>
> (UNDP 1999: 65)

The point is not that people should be satisfied with inferior facilities, but that creative use of what is available can – at least sometimes, at least partially – compensate for them.

Regulatory efforts in areas other than access, though, are proving to be problematic. Most governments are keen to promote electronic commerce, but this requires policies on encryption, and encryption is a political minefield, with commercial and privacy interests ranged against those of law enforcement. Intellectual property is equally resistant to easy solutions. It is difficult to achieve the optimum balance between the protection of authors' rights and the encouragement of widespread access and use of content; for instance, in spring 1999 the European Parliament, to the general derision of the Internet communities, put itself into the strange position of advocating a ban on the temporary caching of Web pages (which conserves bandwidth and speeds access for users) on the grounds that it might make it easier for pirates to steal intellectual property. In any case, even without such problems, the UNDP report points out that tight intellectual property regimes tend to concentrate power in the hands of large corporations and to hinder the efforts of less developed countries to develop an indigenous economic capability (1999: 67–71).

It should be clear that the Internet is not some kind of miraculous force which will in and of itself overcome the many inequalities which exist in the world. But neither is the Internet merely doomed to replicate and reinforce existing patterns of inequality. As an increasingly global, large socio-technical system, the Internet is being shaped by the interplay of social and economic forces around the world as well as by the possibilities and limitations provided by current technologies. Different social groups – academics, librarians, media specialists, commercial interests from various economic sectors, political activists, governments, regulators – view the Internet in different ways and are trying to create spaces within the Internet which serve their own interests. Certainly they do not all have equal power to realise their objectives, and the earlier sections of this chapter have pointed to the hegemonising tendencies of commerce and the implications of this for the maintenance or otherwise of inequalities; commerce is interested in expanding the Internet market only up to the point at which it no longer becomes profitable to pursue expansion.

Perhaps the key feature of the Internet, from the viewpoint of overcoming inequality, is its flexibility. It can contain many different, even contradictory, 'virtual communities': racist organisations use the same infrastructure as the members of the Association of Progressive Communications to spread their messages; anarchists share the same browser software as the financial organisations they are trying to destroy; pornography and sites promoting fundamentalist religions both flourish and are often found together in the vanguard of technical developments. The existence of all these groups, and many others, is not necessarily a good thing, but their presence highlights how the Internet, by being open to further modes of communication and interconnection, can offer scope for policy intervention designed to reduce inequalities.

It may not be possible to stop various developments which have the potential to exacerbate inequality, but it ought to be possible, globally and locally, to work alongside, around and under some of them in order to enlarge the space for widespread access provision, meaningful public discourse, and free or low-cost, high quality information. Access is not the only problem, but with the right kinds of intervention at many levels, problems of access and of the configuration of services and content can begin to be tackled. The Internet is not yet 'for everyone', and is unlikely to be so in the near future, but anything which keeps the Internet open to such a possibility is worth creating or preserving.

NOTES

1 We are grateful to the Virtual Society? Programme of the Economic and Social Research Council which supports the research on which this chapter is based, grant no. L132251050; and to Tiziana Terranova who is working with us on this project but who is not responsible for any of the errors in this chapter.

2 This section is drawn from Thomas and Wyatt (1999) which both explores the development of the Internet, including past alternatives of distributing information globally which have been forgotten or abandoned, and identifies those areas where the future shape of the Internet remains uncertain.

3 For a fuller account of the early history, see Hafner and Lyon (1996). The Internet Society (1999) maintains a collection of Internet histories.

4 The use of the phrase 'stages of development' may be unhelpful as it implies an ordered, even inevitable progression. This is inappropriate because there was no inevitability about the Internet's success or its current structure. During the 1970s and 1980s, both videotex and packet switched data networks appeared to be far more promising as components of a commercial information infrastructure.

5 These data are from the Internet Software Consortium surveys of Internet hosts (1999). These figures provide only approximations of the relative sizes of the sectors. The way in which hosts were counted changed between 1995 and 1998, and the figures do not take account of those hosts (approximately one third in each survey) which use country-specific domain names instead of generic ones and which are more likely to be owned by non-commercial organisations.

6 For a critique of trickle-down, see chapter by Senker, this volume.

7 For an interesting analysis of the relationship between the increased user-friendliness of computers which can empower individual users and the growing corporate power of the companies who design and sell them, see Jordan 1999.

8 This further complicates Internet usage data, because it is likely many of these people will remain in the global statistics about ever-increasing numbers of users.

9 At the time (1992) some of the then existing corporate ISPs argued that by setting the price so low, Demon was undercutting the 'true' market price and – because ISPs would not be able to make profits by charging such low fees – the 'tenner a month' level would actually slow the growth of the access market (Hill 1999: 42).

10 The regulation concerns the division of revenues between telephone companies who initiate and terminate national calls charged at local rates. Essentially, the terminating company receives the lion's share, which is enough to allow it to split the money it receives from the originating company (usually British Telecommunications) with the ISP. Economies of scale, plus other revenue from advertising, premium-rate support services, etc., make it possible (at least in theory) for the ISP to make a profit.

3

PANACEAS AND PROMISES OF DEMOCRATIC PARTICIPATION

Reactions to new channels, from the wireless to the World Wide Web

Rod Allen and Nod Miller

The evangelists and proselytisers who appear with the development of each new information and communications technology usually place democratisation and the reduction of inequality high on the list of benefits that their new technologies are likely to bring about. In 1924, just a year after the British Broadcasting Company was established, its first programme organiser, Caractacus Lewis, set out his views about the potential of the newly-developed wireless for social change. He asked:

> Does it not mean the breakdown of artificial national barriers and the welding of humanity into one composite whole? Does it not mean that each is given a chance to comprehend the significance of national and international affairs, and that all the evils of jealousy and hatred being thus displayed before the world will no longer fester, but be cleansed by the antiseptic of common understanding and common sense?
>
> (Lewis 1924: 144)

Now, more than eighty years later, similar claims are being made for the Internet as it moves towards taking on the status of a mass medium. Rheingold's vision of the implications of the Internet is typical: 'The political significance of CMC [computer-mediated communication] lies in its capacity to challenge the existing political hierarchy's monopoly on powerful communications media, and perhaps thus revitalize citizen-based democracy' (Rheingold 1994: 14).

Radio clearly did not eliminate the evils of international 'jealousy and hatred', as is clear from one world war and countless regional conflicts which have passed by since Caractacus Lewis wrote his book. But it is being argued that there are particular characteristics of the Internet — among them the low cost of entry which makes it an exceptionally economical publishing medium — which heighten the possibility that it might contribute towards the elimination of inequality through its potential for citizen participation.

It seems that as each new media technology emerges, claims are made for its ability to provide enhanced access to information for the mass of the population. It has been argued since the time of Bentham that if people have more information about, for example, political parties or the operation of government, they will be able to participate more effectively in democratic decision-making processes; it is also argued that people who have been offered an abundance of information about their political leaders and structures make better, more responsible citizens and voters. For example, James Mill argued in the 1820s that people could not vote effectively for their political representatives without 'the most perfect knowledge relative to the characters of those who present themselves to their choice ... conveyed freely, and without reserve, from one to another' (Mill 1820/1967: 19). Following this pattern, new technologies are claimed to have a 'democratising' effect, thus leading to the reduction of inequality, at least in terms of the possibility of contributing to the shaping of social change. History shows, however, that such claims are not generally justified, and that new media technologies tend quickly to become dominated either by commercial or state interests.

Inequality in relation to communications media can be seen in terms of ability to receive those media: hence regions have been defined as 'information-poor' (and thus disadvantaged) on the basis of their inability to access communications networks. The problem with this kind of definition is that the ability to operate only as consumers of messages produced by others confers only very limited power; equality in relation to communications media can only be brought about through access to the means of production of media messages. In relation to broadcast media, bandwidth limitations have constrained the possibility of most people ever having access to the airwaves. In the case of the Internet, however, the nature of the technology is such that it is possible for all consumers also to be producers, provided that they have access to a personal computer, some understanding of a simple Web page authoring package and connection to an Internet service provider.

In this chapter, we shall examine some of the claims made when earlier technologies were introduced, focusing particularly on cable television, to gauge the extent to which the promises for democratisation and the reduction of inequality made for those new technologies have been made good, and we shall look at the arguments for and against the possibility of Internet technologies proving to be more effective than their predecessors in contributing to democratisation.

CLAIMS FOR CABLE

Broadcast television is a high-cost medium, and in its early days it was operated without exception either by large, strongly-capitalised commercial corporations or by public authorities. Constrained both by scarcity of broadcast frequencies (which meant that relatively few broadcasters could transmit programmes at the same time) and by the very high cost of plant and production involved, post-war television broadcasting generated widespread debate about its perceived lack of accountability to the public and the lack of accessibility to the airwaves. Broadcasting organisations were seen as gatekeepers, regulating access to the airwaves, reflecting a narrow spectrum of opinion under the guise of consensus and thus excluding many varieties of opinion, taste and interest. It was thought that if the monolithic control of broadcast television as well as the cost of producing programmes could be dealt with, issues of accessibility and accountability might be tackled at the same time (Groombridge 1972).

One hope for overcoming some of these perceived problems was seen in the development of cable television. Cable's history predates that of over-the-air broadcasting; there are remarkable stories of relatively sophisticated cable broadcast systems in

Budapest and Paris at the end of the nineteenth century, transmitting concerts and speech programming over wire to households. But throughout television's first thirty years cable was mainly a passive medium, relaying broadcast signals to homes where television reception was difficult or impossible. This function was most widely developed in North America, where broadcast television stations were only capable of being received inside the geographical area served by a single VHF (or, later, UHF) television transmitter. Viewers living outside the large conurbations, where the largest number of different stations operated, were willing to pay for cable services which imported channels from distant major cities. Inside many cities, the pattern of high-rise development made urban off-air television reception difficult, too, so city apartment-dwellers were also willing to pay for delivery of broadcast signals by cable. There were other reasons for the early development of cable. In Canada, for instance, many people subscribed to cable so that they could watch the US networks' signals, mainly picked up from stations in Buffalo, New York, and distributed in Toronto, because their programmes were thought to be more entertaining than the Canadian national channels; and in northern Europe, cable developed quickly in Belgium and Holland, where polyglot viewers paid to receive broadcast programming in Flemish or Dutch from Belgium and Holland, as well as from Germany, France and Britain.

In Europe, until the beginning of the 1970s, operators of cable networks were forbidden by law to originate programming of their own; their legal function was restricted to that of relaying licensed broadcast programming. But in the United States, Congress took a different view. Cable operators were not merely permitted to produce and transmit cable-only programming; they were actually obliged to offer access to their local channels to anyone who wished to make and transmit programmes, on a first-come first-served basis. Cable services, licensed by the municipalities in which they operated and working under Federal Communications Commission (FCC) rules, made one or more public access channels available according to the number of households they served – the more households, the more channels. Cable services also turned channels over to local school boards, universities and community organisations. This legislative approach was based upon the First Amendment to the Constitution of the United States, which guarantees freedom of speech. But it was quickly seized upon by those who believed that the ability to produce and disseminate television programmes, as well as the ability to receive programmes deriving from a wide variety of different viewpoints, were key issues in the development of participatory democracy. Pimlott's chapter (elsewhere in this book) provides a detailed account of the development of community cable in Canada.

The idea that producing television programmes can of itself address issues of democracy and participation goes back to a number of experiments conducted in the 1950s, particularly those described by Groombridge (1972), which include the Iowa State experiment in Cambridge, Iowa, and the San Bernadino Valley project. In the Iowa experiment, town meetings were televised over the air by Iowa State University's broadcast station WOI-TV, under the title *The Whole Town's Talking*. The US broadcaster and writer Charles Siepmann was involved in the experiment, and he wrote about it at the time:

> When we entered Cambridge we found an apathetic, dispirited community, afraid to discuss its problems. In the past few weeks we have watched a ferment grow in this town. We have watched people as they began to talk about their problems in the open — for the first time. This talk need not, and must not, end with the television programme.
>
> (Siepmann 1952: 66)

In their enthusiasm for the project, neither the normally rigorous Siepmann, who studied early educational broadcasting in the US for UNESCO, nor other contemporary commentators considered the possibility that it was the town meetings themselves, rather than their appearance on television, which might have got the whole town talking.

The second major 1950s experiment, the San Bernadino project, started in 1952 with a grant from the Ford Foundation. Based at San Bernadino Valley College, California, its main objective was the involvement of greater numbers of people in study and development of the communities in that area (Johnson 1956). It was clearly the subject of enormous effort on the part of both educators and broadcasters, and, like the Iowa experiment, it was built around town meetings, which in this case were broadcast over local radio. The project was directed by Eugene Johnson, who went on to adapt the San Bernardino project to television in the form of the Metroplex Project at Washington University, St Louis,

Missouri. Following both radio and television experiments, Johnson is quoted by Groombridge as saying:

> Communication does not take place simply because radio and television programs are broadcast and newspaper printed. The reception of the material offered needs to be organised and its study encouraged ... we need to turn as much time and effort in the task of organising the reception of mass-media offerings as we do to their preparation or broadcast.
>
> (Groombridge 1972: 196)

This again suggests that what is talked about in broadcast town meetings is more important than the fact that they are broadcast, leaving the conclusion that there could have been other kinds of catalysts to wider discussion which might have done much the same job.

However, the idea that dimensions of inequality could be addressed by participatory democracy through television was a powerful one, and it caught the imagination of a number of practitioners and theorists. In a careful historical survey, Hill describes the development of video collectives using the new cable technologies in the early 1970s:

> Most of the early video collectives developed projects which articulated production and reception as essential structural components of their telecommunications visions, reflecting a pragmatic need for new exhibition venues that would accommodate videomakers' aspirations as well as the period's recognition of the politicisation of culture. Specific audience feedback structures were envisioned which exercised portable video's capacity to render real time documentations of everyday events, perceptual investigations, and experimental tech performances.
>
> (Hill 1997)

Another advocate of the power of community video to bring about social change suggests that, 'by using the television set that is in everyone's living room as a forum for community self expression, we may be able to revitalise the democratic dialogue' (Anderson 1975: 68).

Michael Shamberg, now a commercially successful Hollywood producer of pictures such as *The Big Chill*, was an early proselytiser of the democratising and liberating quality of local cable and community television. Shamberg ran a collective called the Raindance Corporation, which was a key component of the New York 'alternative television' movement, and whose activities were based on a belief that the act of producing television programming was in itself democratising. In his 1971 manifesto *Guerrilla Television*, Shamberg writes that,

> Community video will be subversive to any group, bureaucracy or individual which feels threatened by a coalescing of grassroots consciousness. Because not only does decentralised TV serve as an early warning system, it puts people in touch with each other about common grievances.
>
> (Shamberg 1971: 57)

Shamberg visited the UK a number of times as the guest of John Hopkins' Centre for Advanced Television Studies, which was associated with the London Film Cooperative, and energetically proselytised his views to all who would listen. His views carried weight with media activists who were concerned to contribute to community development through media education and training. However, it was commercial interests which led to experiments with local television in Britain. In 1972, the Conservative government gave experimental broadcasting licences to cable television companies in five different localities, allowing them for the first time to originate and to broadcast their own programming on new channels.

British broadcasting policy held universal provision to be of great importance; the objective was that everyone in the country should be able to receive high quality pictures over the air. So once the UK transmitter network reached most of the nation, the need for cable relay diminished. The cable companies, which had invested substantial sums in their networks, needed a new way of persuading customers to pay for cable service, so they petitioned the government to allow them to make and transmit their own programmes, available only to cable subscribers. The experiments took place in Greenwich, Bristol, Sheffield, Swindon and Wellingborough, and the rules set by the government restricted them to locally-originated material. Some of them, such as Maurice Townsend's Greenwich Cablevision, took the form of simple attempts to increase take-up of cable connections by providing local news and interest programming. But others, including notably Swindon Viewpoint and Bristol Channel, set themselves explicit community-oriented missions, and as well as providing local news made an attempt to involve their viewers not only in discussion about local issues but also in the production process.

The experiments were based on flimsy finances, since the operators were neither allowed to fund them through sponsorship or advertising nor permitted to increase cable subscription prices, and by 1975 all but Greenwich and Swindon had collapsed. But in 1975, EMI, the proprietor of Swindon Viewpoint, made a remarkable gesture by handing its ownership and control over to a seven-member board elected at a public meeting attended by some seventy local groups and organisations (Lewis 1978). Funding came from voluntary support and from a local lottery, and Swindon Viewpoint continued for several more years; even so, much of its output was restricted to local news and discussion programmes, and although audience research revealed considerable affection for the service, it was forced first to reduce its hours of transmission, and eventually to close.

In the United States, public access cable quickly fell victim to the undiscriminating nature of the First Amendment: cable operators were not permitted to make distinctions between different kinds of applicants for their public access channels, and as a result most of the attempts at providing alternative public service material were swamped by a combination of wannabe television stars, religious revivalists and pornographers. Most cable subscribers in Manhattan, for instance, associate public access channels with a performer called Ugly George, who was indeed a user of small-format video equipment of the kind so enthusiastically embraced by Michael Shamberg. He used it to compile a weekly programme in which he stalked the streets of New York asking young women to take their clothes off in front of his portable video camera. The show ran for more than ten years.

It remained true that alternative television distribution technologies survived and thrived in the market because they offered programming which was not available on the air. In 1975, Home Box Office (HBO), now owned by Time-Warner, bought exclusive television rights to 'The Thriller in Manila', the heavyweight championship fight which established Muhammed Ali's reputation, and offered it exclusively to cable viewers. HBO followed this up with its pay-movie concept, through which cable viewers can subscribe to channels providing recent films. Today, there is a plethora of cable-only channels whose audiences in aggregate now exceed viewership of network television, although shares of audience for individual channels remain relatively small. Some of these cable channels have dimensions of, or pretensions to, alternative or public service television; Cable News Network (CNN), Black Entertainment Television and some family-oriented channels like USA Network address audiences who are not served by on-air networks or local stations.

Paradoxically, though, the main providers of public service television – the network of stations which make up the Public Broadcasting Service – remain firmly in the on-air domain, using the channels reserved for them (and from which commercial broadcasters were excluded) in the 1960s by the Federal Communications Commission. Cable's main contribution to television has been to extend somewhat the frontiers of traditional television forms like soap and situation comedy, with programmes like HBO's *Larry Sanders Show, Sex in the City* and *The Sopranos*. There are channels devoted to factual programming, such as the Discovery Channel, but a surprisingly large proportion of their output is devoted to military subjects or wildlife and cannot be considered to be a significant extension to on-air provision. On the other hand, most commentators would acknowledge that the development of twenty-four hour news, music and sport services, such as Cable News Network (CNN), Music Television (MTV) and Eastern Sports Programming Network (ESPN) represented valuable, if modest, additions to the totality of US television. However, none of these developments addressed issues of local democratisation or empowerment. On the contrary, the reason they have attracted business investment is because they are effective in maintaining levels of cable subscription.

In Britain, broadcasting was effectively deregulated in the mid-1980s, with legislation that made it possible to set up satellite channels intended for reception by British audiences. But the local access and participation experiments of the 1970s were forgotten, as British satellite broadcasters merely copied the US formula – or, in some cases, imported it wholesale (we have our own Discovery Channel, our own MTV and our own sports and news channels). A narrow range of choice was extended, but the real frontiers of television broadcasting remained the property of terrestrial on-air broadcasters like BBC2 and Channel 4.

None of this should come as a surprise. The financial investments involved in providing new cable and satellite services are enormous. Small operators, like Greenwich Cablevision or the original, pre-Murdoch, owners of Sky Television, were almost instantly squeezed out by very large media conglomerates, many of whom were also major players in terrestrial television. Their profits lay in the mass distribution of inexpensive programming, not in focused, local, hand-tailored material which reached out into specific communities. If football fans can be said to have represented an under-served community, then the development of the Premiere League for BSkyB could conceivably be seen as a community service. But even such gestures to minority audiences as Sky Scottish, a two-hour nightly news and current affairs service intended for Scottish viewers, proved unprofitable and were closed quickly. Ordinary citizens have no more access to the airwaves than they did in the early 1970s, when the BBC Community Programmes Unit and LWT's *Look Here*, produced by one of the authors of this chapter, went out seeking viewers to participate in 'access' programme-making. The alternative distribution technology, which may have held considerable promise as a democratising or empowering vehicle, was swiftly and comprehensively hi-jacked by commercial interests, to the exclusion of non-commercial possibilities. Even the most recent technological developments in digital distribution have produced very few proposals to return to communities of interest or geographical commonality for programming opportunities: digital television, too, makes best economic sense when used for mass delivery.

One of the main problems with television is that however small the audience, and however compact and miniaturised the technology, it is still expensive to produce and distribute. When a medium demands significant and continuing cash investment, it is in the interests of those who already have significant investments in that medium or similar media to keep the costs of entry high and thus to discourage new entrants who, they fear, will dilute the market. This is done in television at least partly by the setting of standards of spending on programmes – 'professional' standards which involve highly-paid actors, technicians and producers – which in its turn requires entrants to the market to match those standards in order to attract audiences. It may also be argued that television as we know it is labour- and capital-intensive, requiring human, technical, journalistic and creative input at some cost; this, too, excludes small entrepreneurs and those whose motivations are not commercial.

CLAIMS FOR THE WORLD WIDE WEB

The most recent technology – the World Wide Web – does not require actors, camerapeople, writers, producers and tons of equipment. The cost of entry to the Web can be astonishingly low when compared to its predecessor technologies. Anyone with access to a computer, an internet service provider (ISP) and some very basic authoring software can become a Web publisher in a matter of hours. (Thomas and Wyatt, in this volume, consider some further issues related to the growth of and access to the Web). There is literally no cost of distribution, because it is the user of a Web site, not its publisher, who is responsible for the transfer of information from remote to local computer. Moreover, a number of authors have taken up the idea that the Web exhibits many of the characteristics of the forum of public discussion and interchange described by Habermas as the public sphere (1989; 1990), and thus may have considerable democratising potential.

The public sphere is seen as a component in the process of representative democracy, and the discussion and interchange which is involved is thought to be at least as important as the actual decisions or policies that arise. The idea of a space for public discussion in which all participants had the equal right to be heard is closely allied to notions of Athenian democracy, and Habermas identifies its development in modern times in the coffee houses of seventeenth and eighteenth century London, where issues of the day were discussed by those with time and resources to do so. By the nineteenth century, he argues, public opinion, formed by rational-critical debate, had become the 'officially designated discussion partner' of parliament (Habermas 1989). The concept of the public sphere has been invoked in discussions of the public service dimension of radio and television broadcasting (see for example Garnham 1986a, Dahlgren 1995). However, postmodernist writers such as Lyotard (1984) argue that to conceive of the public sphere as defined by Habermas to be operating in television broadcasting is to affirm the dominant Establishment 'metanarrative' and to ignore pluralities of opinion in society. Moreover, structural changes in broadcasting in recent years have diminished the broadcasting organisations' public responsibilities, and in the recent era of deregulation and privatisation it has become harder and harder to identify Habermas's 'discursive arena' in today's television and radio.

But the debate about the extent of the public sphere's space in today's press, radio and television has not discouraged the enthusiastic adoption of the Internet as an ideal site for Habermasian public discourse. Writers such as Negroponte (1995), Poster (1995), Ess (1994), Langham (1994), Gaynor (1997) and many others seize on the disintermediated nature of the Internet as providing unfettered access for open and rapid exchange of opinions between individuals, and hence the conditions required for the 'discursive arena' that Habermas described.

Habermas suggested that in order for a public sphere of the kind he identified to flourish, it should conform to certain conditions. These were:

> Every subject with the competence to speak and act is allowed to take part in a discourse;
> Everyone is allowed to question any assertion whatever;
> Everyone is allowed to introduce any assertion whatever into the discourse;
> Everyone is allowed to express his/her attitudes, desires and needs;
> No speaker may be prevented, by internal or external coercion, from exercising the rights laid down above.
>
> (Habermas 1990: 86)

This is a formulation which not only describes the rights which can be exercised by a Web publisher, but also accurately defines the conditions under which the unmoderated newsgroups on the Internet operate. Internet enthusiasts argue that the interaction which is possible between Net users is unconstrained by power relations. Rheingold talks of 'the great equaliser [which] can equalise the balance of power between citizens and power barons' (1991: 6). Grossman sees a radical change in the nature of political communication:

> The big losers in the present-day reshuffling and resurgence of public influence are the traditional institutions that have served as the main intermediaries between government and its citizens – the political parties, labor unions, civic associations, even the commentators and correspondents in the mainstream press.
>
> (Grossman 1995: 16)

Others, though, take a more dystopian view. Leggewie observes that many of the potential benefits of 'netizenship' are not being taken up:

> Like television, cyberspace is being turned into a central-
> ised marketplace; the inherent potential for horizontal,
> two-way communication (which is more pronounced than
> television) is being ignored, thus remaining unused and
> underdeveloped. As a result, the Internet is falling far short
> both of its potential for a "digital participatory democ-
> racy" and even the ambivalent achievements of
> "teledemocracy".
>
> (Leggewie 1997)

McChesney, in his analysis of the history of US communications policymaking and its implications for the Internet, is not compre-hensively dystopian, but he takes a more cautious view than those who unreservedly define the Internet as a democratising, liberating public space. He acknowledges that 'newly-developed computer and digital communications can undermine the ability to control communication in a traditionally hierarchical manner' (1996: 109). But he believes that much of the Internet, and the policymaking surrounding it, has already been given over to large corporations whose interests lie away from the creation of opportunities for public discussion. Nevertheless, because of the low costs and technical ease of entry to the Internet, he suggests that there is an important segment of Internet users whose inter-ests do lie in developing opportunities for 'informed, interactive debate':

> Even if the market is permitted to determine the course of
> the information highway and there is minimal public
> deliberation over fundamental communication policy
> issues, there is no evidence that the Internet, or the subse-
> quent information highway, can possibly come under the
> same sort of monopoly corporate control as have broad-
> casting and traditional media ... the key issue is whether
> the non-profit, non-commercial sector of cyberspace will
> be able to transform our societies radically for the better
> and to do so without fundamental policy intervention. In
> short, will this sector be able to create a 21st-century,
> Habermasian "public sphere", where informed interactive

debate can flower independent of government or commercial control? This follows the critical strain of democratic theory that argues that the structural basis for genuine democratic communication lies with a media system free from the control of either the dominant political or economic powers of the day.

(McChesney 1996: 108)

Over the past three years, the World Wide Web dimension of the Internet has been wholeheartedly adopted by industry and commerce as a new marketing communications medium, and, as Morris and Ogan (1996) and many others argue, it is taking on many of the characteristics of a 'traditional' mass medium.

CONCLUSION

There are currently (mid-1999) more than 200 million pages on the World Wide Web. Many of them are hosted by big international corporations who see the Web as another great competitive marketing space like television or the press. Although the business model is not yet settled, electronic commerce (e-commerce – the sale of goods to consumers through the Web) is becoming a very significant business sector, and in a few short years the Web has become a normative dimension of most corporations' advertising, marketing and public relations activities. Other major companies are struggling to find dominant positions as information and entertainment providers on the Web, from the BBC (http://www.bbc.co.uk) and Cable News Network (http://www.cnn.com) to Microsoft with its content-rich sites in a wide range of market sectors (http://www.msn.com). Yet at the same time the Web carries full unmediated texts of key documents, from the Starr Report on the impeachment of President Clinton to the Fryer Report on lifelong learning, and many millions of pages, carrying many millions of different opinions, published by many millions of individuals. The difference, of course, is that the big corporations can use traditional marketing techniques and investments to draw attention to their sites, whereas individuals can only hope that their pages are found through search engines or link-swaps with like-minded publishers.

The Internet has not even reached the stage at which cable television could be found at the beginning of the 1970s. As one of us has argued at length elsewhere, it is 'still a chimera in cyberspace; it has been going for a shorter period of time than the cinema had been going when D.W. Griffith discovered parallel action, and so the Internet's final form is, to say the least, yet to be determined' (Allen 1999: 93). Whether the Web is more likely to be seen through the television screen than the computer monitor, and how information and entertainment provided through the Web are finally to be paid for are among the many issues that will not be settled for years to come.

Until now, freedom of access to the Internet has been reasonably widespread, although while Africa still has less than a million connections 'widespread' will remain a relative term. It has certainly been colonised by business and government, but unlike the great empires of the nineteenth century the Internet offers infinite landscape; there is in practical terms no limit to the number of pages that can be published. So unlike broadcasting, whose history can in many ways be analysed as a territorial struggle between corporate behemoths all of whom wanted to colonise the same space, the Internet may be able to accommodate all kinds of needs and uses. But publishing needs readers (or, in computer language, users), and there is a finite limit to the amount of time any one individual can spend surfing the Web.

What needs to be monitored carefully as the Net grows is the way in which users choose how to use it. If people use their time in front of the screen primarily to play games such as *Doom* or *Mortal Kombat,* to engage in chat-room talk about sex or to do tele-shopping, then yet again the promise of enhanced democratic participation through the new medium is hardly likely to be fulfilled.

4

PUBLIC SERVICE BROADCASTING AND NEW DISTRIBUTION TECHNOLOGIES

Issues of equality, access and choice in the transactional television environment

Kathy Walker

The launch of Sky TV's interactive service on its Sports Extra channel in August 1999 was described variously in the press as a 'new broadcasting dawn', 'the brave new world of interactive' (Battersby 1999), and 'television history being made' (Cleveland-Peck and Hammersley 1999[1]). The occasion for the launch of this new interactive service was the Premiership football match between Arsenal and the European and FA cup holders Manchester United. Facilitated by the additional channels available on the new digital system, viewers were able to select an alternative camera angle of the game, view action replays and highlights, and call up match statistics, all while watching the live coverage of the match. This event and the hyperbole surrounding it are not unusual in the sense of euphoria they convey about technological change in the media sector. They also illustrate in a number of ways the wider issues of choice, control, access and exclusion, which are central to debates about the implications of the current market-driven broadcasting environment. The selection of Premiership football as the launch pad for the development of interactive services is not surprising in view of the importance of exclusive sports coverage to the sustained development of satellite television. The interactive service complements both existing subscription and pay-TV strategies and provides effective promotion for Sky's new digital service. Additionally, claims that for the first time in Britain viewers were able to *choose* what they watched of the match and to *control* how they watched it are indicative of the promises made in respect of the benefits of new communication technologies and the competitive broadcasting environment in which they are developing. These claims are questionable on a number of grounds, not least because the service is available only to Sky digital subscribers who in addition pay a £25 minimum monthly payment to receive the three-channel Sky sports package.

In the last two decades broadcasting organisations in the UK and Europe more generally have undergone considerable structural and regulatory change largely the result, as McQuail points out, of new technological possibilities, mediated by policy and politics (McQuail 1990: 313). The development of broadband cable and Direct Broadcast by Satellite (DBS) opened up a wide range of options for television delivery, presenting opportunities to challenge the rationale for regulation and public service broadcasting based on spectrum scarcity, and facilitating the expansion of media conglomerates eager to develop new markets for programming, advertising and pay-TV. The process of deregulation and liberalisation of broadcasting structures in the UK culminated with the 1990 Broadcasting Act which opened the way for a relaxation of public service obligations in the Independent Television sector and facilitated the development of a more commercial, market-driven television environment generally. Continuing this process, the 1996 Broadcasting Act set out the structures and conditions for the development of digital services on the competing commercial platforms of terrestrial, cable and satellite television.

Attitudes and responses to the process of liberalisation and deregulation in policy documents, academic accounts and the media itself have tended to become polarised. Proponents of broadcasting as a public service, with its clear commitments to universality and equality in terms of access and range of programming, have argued that an increasingly commercialised broadcasting environment reduces the range and choice of programming available and discriminates between audiences on the grounds of income. Golding in particular has drawn attention to this inequality of access to cultural goods which, 'sharply differentiate between groups unequally located in the market economy' (Golding 1990: 90). In contrast, arguments for a liberalised, market-led broadcasting environment have consistently criticised the lack of accountability and elitism of public service broadcasting, maintaining that market mechanisms provide the best framework for the expansion of radio and television, the promotion of greater competition and opportunity in the provision of programming, and a wider range of choice for audiences.

This polarity of positions reflected in numerous accounts of the changing broadcasting environment is somewhat simplistic, as Curran and Seaton's account of the policy making process makes clear (Curran and Seaton 1997: 331–57). The focus of this chapter, however, is to investigate the ways in which the overall thrust of change has impacted on the perception and understanding of the role and purposes of broadcasting and to assess the implication of these changes for audiences. As market forces increasingly dictate the structures of broadcasting in the UK, this chapter examines the way equality is conceptualised in traditional approaches to broadcasting as a public service and contrasts this with the very different definition of equality employed in the discourses of market-led systems and encapsulated in terms such as 'consumer sovereignty'. Each system claims to offer a better service for audiences as a whole but employs very different understandings of the role of broadcasting and the relationship between broadcaster and audience. Conflicting interpretations of issues of choice and access also underpin the ways in which perceptions of equality and inequality are constructed within the discourses and policy of each approach. By examining the development of cable and satellite technologies and the rhetoric surrounding them, this chapter looks critically at the claims of extended choice and diversity in the multi-channel television environment. It explores the ways in which decisions taken at the policy-making stage frame the context in which these technologies develop and shape the nature of the benefits they provide for audiences. The traditional public service approach to broadcasting offers universal access to a wide range of quality programming with the aim of raising cultural standards and providing a forum for democratic discussion and debate. The new communication technologies of cable and satellite, which underpin the market-driven, commercial environment, it is suggested, will empower the consumer and maximise individual choice, but it is choice through exclusion, predicated increasingly on the ability to pay directly for the services provided. This chapter will examine the tensions apparent between these competing claims and consider the likelihood that income inequalities will play an increasing part in determining access to television services leading to greater social inequity.

PUBLIC SERVICE BROADCASTING

Until the 1980s, despite their very different national and cultural features, all broadcasting systems in western Europe had included some public service element in their arrangements. Blumler and Nossiter's typology of broadcasting systems, based on the balance of their relations to public/political and market forces, identified the UK as a mixed system with strong public service regulation overall (Blumler and Nossiter 1991: 407). Although the BBC is most readily identified as the main public service provider, public service ideals and expectations extended across the whole range of broadcasting outputs. In effect, until 1990, both the public broadcaster, the BBC, and the independent sector, comprising the ITV network and Channel 4, were strictly regulated in terms of programme content and quality. The limited number of channels available for broadcasting, referred to as 'spectrum scarcity', had initially been a factor in the carefully controlled development of television services. However, technical constraints were not the only factors shaping attitudes towards broadcasting. Central to the ethos of public service broadcasting in the UK has been the conviction that broadcasting should be directed towards the public good rather than private gain. As Keane has argued, 'the media should be for the public use and enjoyment of all citizens and not for the private gain or profit of political rulers or businesses' (Keane 1991: XII). Garnham has also challenged accounts which justify public service broadcasting solely on the grounds of frequency scarcity and which have formed the basis of a range of economic arguments for abandoning public service commitments as restrictions on frequencies have diminished. He argues that the justification for publicly regulated television is more complex and,

> lies in its superiority to the market as a means of providing all citizens, whatever their wealth or geographical location, equal access to a wide range of high-quality

entertainment, information and education, and as a means of ensuring that the aim of the programme producer is the satisfaction of a range of audience tastes rather than only those that show the largest profit.

(Garnham 1990: 120)

Underlying the more detailed codes and regulatory practices of public service broadcasting, therefore, is a clear sense of the role and responsibility of broadcasters to their audiences. The principle of universality is a clear commitment to the belief that broadcasting should be available equally to all citizens, irrespective of income or geographical location. This principle has underpinned both the structures of production and transmission and the funding mechanism of the broadcasting networks. The fact that the BBC and ITV sectors competed for audiences and not for income is widely acknowledged as an important element in producing the broad range of quality programming associated with British television. During the 1980s the BBC licence fee was the focus of criticism from politicians and free market economists who argued that it was a form of regressive taxation which insulated the BBC from direct competition resulting in inefficiencies, high costs and restrictive practices. However, it has many advantages as a means of ensuring equality of access to high quality broadcast services. It provides a steady source of income for the production of quality programming as, unlike more general forms of government taxation and advertising, all income goes directly to the BBC and it does not discriminate on grounds of income or the cost of the service provided to the individual. The fee also helps to insulate the broadcaster from the vested interests of advertisers, corporate investors and government. It has continued to provide the simplest method of funding for a universal, non-transactional medium and is the 'ultimate enabler of the whole system, for a total service within which a large element of financial redistribution is entailed' (Smith 1986: 5).

The principle of universal provision also has a further dimension. Although the ideas and aspirations of public service broadcasting have changed and evolved over time, universality has always implied that broadcast services should be for the benefit of the public as a whole and should therefore provide access to a wide range and diversity of programming suitable for all interests and tastes. Underlying these aims is the fundamental assumption they embody about the social and cultural purposes of broadcasting and the recognition of the importance of the structures and ethos of broadcasting in reflecting and shaping society. Central to the goals defined by the first Director General of the BBC, John Reith, was the belief that broadcasting should be challenging and require active participation rather than passive absorption. From the earliest days of radio, broadcasting as a public service was organised on the principle that programmes should educate, inform and entertain the public, 'forcing it to confront the frontiers of its own taste' (Smith quoted in Kumar 1986: 59). This policy of mixed programming provides diversity and choice for audiences and was designed to satisfy different needs and sections of society. Broadcasting was seen as a means of both extending individual horizons and of reflecting national interests and the cultural traditions of audiences. The role of the BBC as producer and commissioner of original programming in music, drama and the arts has been of central importance to the direction of cultural production and consumption in Britain. In addition, services received universally throughout the whole country gave audiences a source of shared interest and inclusion in major cultural experiences (Cardiff and Scannell 1987). The commitment to universality and mixed programming therefore implies that some measure of equality is achieved on the basis that the parameters of choice and access are the same for everyone irrespective of economic or social position.

The commitment to the provision of a broadcasting service responsible not only to individual listeners and viewers but to the collective interest of society as a whole is central to understanding the concept of equality embedded in public service discourse. This commitment is reflected not only in the social and cultural purposes of public service broadcasting but also in its contribution to the development and maintenance of an active democratic culture. Equal access to a wide range of universally available information and diversity of opinions is recognised as essential to the democratic process (Garnham 1986, Livingstone and Lunt 1994, O'Malley 1994).[2] The broadcaster's role as a source of information and forum of debate is an essential contribution to the creation of a public space for the free market of ideas and opinions. Scannell has demonstrated that the democratic thrust of broadcasting was established by early radio in the way 'it equalised public life through the common access it established for all members of society' (Scannell 1990: 16). Garnham describes the public service model of broadcasting as 'the embodiment of the principles of the public sphere' (Garnham 1986: 31) a concept identified by Habermas to represent a realm of social life in which public opinion is formed and access is guaranteed for all citizens (Habermas 1979).

It is important to note here that notions of equality implicit in the cultural, social and political traditions of public service broadcasting derive from this recognition of the audience as citizens and 'participants in the great affairs of the nation' (Curran and Seaton 1997: 303). There is an essential difference between value systems and social relations sustained by communication systems in public and private ownership (Garnham 1990; Ang 1991). The perception of the *audience-as-public* in comparison to the *audience-as-market* is reflected in attitudes to programming and scheduling and underpins the sense of responsibility to the audience beyond the demands of a purely market relationship. In terms of programme content, this has largely implied the provision of a diverse, informative and enriching range of productions rather than only that which attracts a mass audience. This concept of the audience as citizen, and the responsibilities it implies, is central to the formation and affirmation of audience expectations regarding programming. As Blumler and Nossiter's research has shown, these constructions of the audience member lead to presumptions about the type of programming they prefer: 'a system that is entertainment-dominated tends to presume that viewers are not normally looking for deeper involvement' (Blumler and Nossiter 1991: 413). In a predominantly market system, audiences are addressed as consumers not only of the programmes they consume but also the products advertised alongside them.

This analysis of the construction and embodiment of notions of equality in the concept of public service broadcasting suggests an idealistic view of British broadcasting in the early 1980s. However, the BBC and the BBC/ITV duopoly were subject to a range of criticism, which suggested a less than satisfactory achievement of these aims. The cultural role of the BBC, in particular, has been criticised as elitist, with audiences having little say in the range of programming offered to them and little opportunity to broaden the spectrum of society represented on screen. Criticisms of lack of accountability and representative structures could be said to undermine the notions of choice and access, which are fundamental components of the public service model of equality. However, as Keane has cautioned, it is important not to confuse the values and goals of public service broadcasting with existing public service institutions and their limitations (Keane 1991: 11). Public service broadcasting is a concept which has evolved over time. Its structures and practices have adapted to, and been strengthened by, its response to changing social conditions and pressures from government, audiences and programme-makers. As Garnham points out, 'public service broadcasting has, like all the endeavours of fallible humans, a flawed record. But as an ideal it has certainly not failed' (Garnham 1989: 33).

In the 1980s however, a new concept of broadcasting with a very different value system and perception of access and choice challenged the public service model. These developments will be examined more fully in the following section.

CONSUMER SOVEREIGNTY AND THE FREE MARKET

A number of developments occurred in the 1980s which led to what has been described as a crisis in the ethos of public service broadcasting and the rise to dominance of a new philosophy of the competitive market and consumer choice. Pressures for deregulation (the relaxation of rules or regulation with a light touch), and liberalisation (the introduction of competition into a previously monopolistic or oligopolistic environment) led to major changes in the British broadcasting environment, reflecting, as Collins points out, 'a waning of confidence in state and parastatal agencies and waxing confidence in competition and the market as allocative agencies' (Collins 1990: 99). The pressure for deregulation and liberalisation was partly in response to the new technologies of cable and DBS which presented new ways of delivering television and offered new methods of charging the audience for programming via subscription and pay-per-view. The changes also reflected a new political dynamic with a neo-liberal emphasis on free enterprise, market competition and anti-statist policies. Thus the themes of privatisation and competitive markets underpinned the changing political initiatives towards broadcasting and linked them to policies of economic regeneration and technological innovation.

Government policy towards the development of broadband cable was the first sign of a significant change in political philosophy towards broadcasting. Until 1980, as Negrine notes, any change in the conditions under which cable operated had been made largely with the intention of integrating it into existing structures of broadcasting (Negrine 1988: 23).[3] The report of the 1982

Information Technology Advisory Panel (ITAP), however, put forward the more radical arguments of the pro-cable lobby, suggesting that,

> More space should make access to television easier, resulting in a more 'democratic' use of the medium. Moreover, the new channels ought to react more accurately than existing services to the viewing preferences of their audiences as a direct result of the activities of the market.
>
> (Hollins 1984: 61)

The ITAP report reflected the growing confidence in the ability of information and communication technologies (ICTs) to boost economic growth and generate employment, and resonated with the rhetoric of new opportunity and choice in the provision of cable television. ITAP set the character of discussion for the subsequent Hunt Committee (Home Office 1982) and, in 1984, the Cable and Broadcasting Act enabled the widespread, entertainment-led development of cable systems, privately funded by revenue from popular programming channels.

Policy for the development of a UK DBS initiative reflected many of the characteristics of the discussion around cable although, in the case of DBS, they were underpinned by international regulations on frequencies, orbital slots and technical specifications, as well as European agreements on broadcasting standards. The licence for the initial Direct Broadcast satellite project was awarded to the BBC in 1984 but, due to complex problems, mainly linked to the cost of the British-built satellite stipulated by the government, the BBC were forced to abandon the scheme (Negrine 1989: 224). The franchise was later awarded to a private consortium, British Satellite Broadcasting (BSB). BSB finally launched their service in April 1990, despite delays arising from the escalating costs associated with using a high-powered satellite specified by international regulation, problems with reception equipment, and the need to transmit using a new high definition broadcasting standard defined by the CEC. Delays in the launch of the service were to prove critical, however, since News Corporation's Sky service had been launched some months earlier from the Luxembourg-based Astra satellite. With a head-start in the market and none of the technical constraints imposed on BSB, Sky proved more adept in both the standards and public relations battles. In November 1990, just after the Broadcasting Bill became statute,

BSB was ignominiously merged with Sky. Despite widespread concern, the government took the line that market forces should prevail and chose not to refer the merger to the Monopolies and Mergers Commission (Chippindale and Franks 1991).

In 1986, the Committee on Financing the BBC, known as the Peacock Committee, applied a stringent economic approach towards broadcasting policy where previously discussion had been in predominantly social and cultural terms. The committee was originally set up to examine the financing of the BBC but extended its brief to consider the whole structure and regulation of broadcasting. The key principle at the heart of the Peacock report was that broadcasting was an economic activity which should be provided on a competitive basis unless there were compelling reasons not to do so (Veljanowski 1989: IX). Its approach assumed that the public service model exemplified by the BBC had produced an overprotected, stultified and unresponsive broadcasting system and, if this was to change, it should be consumers and programme providers interacting in a free market who decided on programming. A more competitive broadcasting system, responsive to consumer demands, would produce greater diversity and choice. Peacock marked a break with the traditional view of the role of broadcasting summed up by its central finding that,

> British broadcasting should move towards a sophisticated market system based on consumer sovereignty. That is a system which recognises that viewers and listeners are the best ultimate judges of their own interest, which they can best satisfy if they have the option of purchasing the broadcasting services they require from as many alternative sources of supply as possible.
>
> (Home Office 1986: para.592)

The notion of consumer sovereignty was not seen as incompatible with the concept of broadcasting as a public service. However, in contrast to the comprehensive model of public service broadcasting which underpinned the approach to broadcasting as a whole, the new model interpreted public service broadcasting merely as a necessary 'modification of purely commercial provision' to ensure the production of programming which commercial providers would have little incentive to supply (para 580).

Although a number of Peacock's recommendations originally found little favour, debate about broadcasting issues became increasingly dominated by economic arguments and the language of market competition and consumer choice. This was reflected in the 1988 White Paper entitled, *Broadcasting in the 90s: Competition, Choice and Quality*. By the time the Broadcasting Bill was enacted by parliament, the policy-making process ensured that the broadcasting environment had been irrevocably opened up to the market and to the rigours of commercial competition. For the first time, the independent sector became subject to competitive tendering, with ITV franchises allocated on the basis of a financial bid, albeit one which had to meet a quality threshold. Channel 4 competed with ITV for advertising revenue and all broadcasters were required to commission 25 per cent of their programming from independent producers. The Act also established an even more liberalised, market-led framework for the developing cable and satellite industries with no positive programme obligations or requirements for diversity on cable and satellite channels. In addition, there was no longer any requirement for local programming in the licensing conditions for cable, a commitment that had been a cornerstone of earlier policy. In response to intense lobbying from the cable industry during the passage of the Broadcasting Bill, restrictions on foreign ownership of cable franchises were formally removed, plans to separate delivery and retailing of services were abandoned, and a technology-neutral environment was established to promote growth.

Thus a very different view of the role and aims of broadcasting have, to a large extent, reshaped the broadcasting environment of the 1990s. The Conservative government's philosophy of 'rolling back the state' and minimising the regulation of broadcast services has relegated the public service ethos to a small proportion of the overall television sector. As a result of the 1990 Broadcasting Act, since 1993 only the BBC and Channel 4 have been required to broadcast programmes as a public service (Department of National Heritage 1992: 14, para. 3.5), with the independent sector subject to regulation with a light touch. Cable and satellite channels, although licensed by the Independent Television Commission (ITC), are not subject to positive programming requirements. The explicit social and cultural aims and requirements of public service broadcasting are largely absent from the competitive broadcasting environment which responds essentially to economic and market imperatives.

In this model, the concept of equality and the claims for democratisation of broadcasting structures are based on the rights and opportunities of the individual rather than a commitment to the collective benefit of society as a whole. Instead of a menu of mixed programming determined by the broadcasters, individual citizens, now referred to as consumers, have the freedom to make their own choice of programming from the wide array of options available in the market system. More channels provide not only more programming but also a wider source of programming and a more democratic use of the television medium. Consumers are freed from the narrow confines imposed by existing broadcast structures to express their own individual choices and preferences from the diverse range and variety of programming available. In the multi-channel environment, the *internal diversity* of mixed programming on a single channel is replaced by *external diversity* where 'individual channels become less mixed in their programming and differentiate themselves from each other with a strong and consistent "brand image"' (Collins 1990: 95). The increasing fragmentation of society into different social, cultural and economic groups, it is argued, has made it increasingly difficult for the mixed programming schedules of existing broadcasters to satisfy the variety of tastes existing in these groups. This reflects Toffler's view of the fragmentation of the mass audience served by national broadcasting systems and the move to 'narrow-casting to specialised audience segments' (Toffler 1980: 171–83). Specialist thematic channels are therefore better able to meet the needs of a diverse, multi-cultural society and to represent the widening range of social and political outlooks. To a large extent, these views also embody the philosophy and imperatives of specialised production and consumption evident in other areas of the market economy and reinforce the concept of programming as a product or commodity.

The market system, and the new technologies on which it is based, also redefine the relationship between the audience and the programme provider. The exercise of consumer choice establishes a more direct link between the audience and the new channels and should ensure that programme services are more responsive to consumer preference rather than the broadcaster or advertiser's perception of audience tastes. This closer relationship is facilitated by the technical properties of cable, DBS and the new digital services which enable the programming to be encrypted and made available only to subscribers. The universal licence fee and advertising have been the most effective means of funding broadcasting indirectly because of its essential properties as a 'public good', defined by Hills as 'goods held in common, paid for in common, accessed by all and benefiting everyone' (Hills 1991: 3). Broadcasting exhibits the two essential properties of public goods: firstly, that it is very difficult, if not impossible, to exclude non-payers from its benefits and secondly, its benefits are not reduced by extra users. The transactional environment of cable, DBS and new digital services is, in contrast, predicated on the technical capacity to encrypt the signals they distribute. In order to receive the current analogue services for cable and BSkyB and the new digital television services, consumers need a 'conditional access system', commonly known as the set-top box. This performs two key functions: firstly, it receives and unscrambles encrypted signals and secondly, it manages subscription, pay-per-view and the delivery of the programming paid for. For this reason, it has been likened to 'the electronic turnstile in the set-top box' which makes pay-TV possible. This technology enables audiences to make their opinions and choices known directly by either paying or not paying for particular channels or pay-per-view events.

RHETORIC AND REALITY

As the earlier discussion has suggested, it is possible to identify a gap between the discourse and reality of public service broadcasting and its contribution to notions of equality. It would be unwise to ignore pro-market arguments that focus on the potential of new channels to give the public the greater choice they want since, as Keane has argued, this overlooks 'the ways in which the alleged "balance", "quality" standards and universalism of existing public service media are routinely perceived by certain audiences as "unrepresentative"' (Keane 1992: 122). Similarly, although cable and satellite channels are widely criticised for their overtly entertainment-based format and lack of quality programming, it is difficult to dismiss the very real attraction of entertainment to audiences. Audiences' predilection for entertainment is not new as is evidenced by the BBC's acknowledgement of the need to increase the amount of light entertainment in its schedules following the introduction of independent television in the 1950s. For the BBC, this illustrates the 'fundamental contradiction between the wish to edify the audience on the one hand and the need to attract the audience on the other' (Ang 1991: 110–13).

With this in mind, however, this chapter will now turn to the similar, if not vastly greater, gap between the rhetoric and reality of the deregulated market-led environment. It will examine how far policies of competition, and the technologies on which they rely, have lived up to promises of providing greater access and choice for audiences. It will also address research which suggests that the introduction of market principles and commercial approaches are contributing to even greater inequalities of access to information and entertainment due to the transactional nature of their availability and the increasingly negative impacts of commercial and competitive influences on programme and service provision.

The concept of equality premised on notions of choice and access in the deregulated, market-led broadcasting environment, is problematic in a number of senses. Whilst the independent influence of technology in enabling and constraining social choices has to be taken into account, the emphasis on technology-driven change tends to overemphasise the democratising potentials of the technology. As the earlier discussion has indicated, new communication technologies, and the level of expectation surrounding them underpinned the wave of deregulation and commercialisation of broadcasting structures which took place in Europe in the 1980s. Most explanations of the policy-making process for cable and satellite emphasise that strategies to foster the economic and industrial potentials of these technologies over-rode the more cultural considerations of broadcasting policy (Hills 1991). More dramatically, Negrine (1988) has suggested that the acquiescence of European governments allowed the technological rollercoaster to move unobstructed by political and social consequences. It is clear that policy decisions in these areas were significantly influenced by the technologically determinist views of politicians, governments and corporations that new information and communication technologies were capable of dramatically re-shaping national and international markets, the media environment and society in general. The identification of cable and satellite with the UK government's information technology strategies stressed their potential for industrial and economic expansion and the generation of economic and employment benefits. A very similar rhetoric underpins current debates about convergence and digital technologies in the national and European context. This desire to jump on the bandwagon of technological change, however, belies the importance of key political and corporate actors in shaping the direction and development of change.

Thus, although it is possible to dispute the level to which

broadcasting policy was subsumed by industrial strategy, it is evident that the language of the market, competition and expansion were assimilated into a policy arena previously dominated by cultural considerations. Hills has argued that government policies which focus predominantly on accelerating the pace of technological change and restructuring markets to encourage large-scale private investment consistently ignore citizens' needs (Hills 1991). Private commercial interests are prioritised in the interests of technological development and competitive advantage. The more recent Green Paper, *Convergence of the Telecommunications, Media and Information Technology Sectors* (CEC 1997b) is underpinned by a similar industry perspective, and presents a technologically determinist message that convergence will inevitably lead to greater liberalisation of the audio-visual sector. Research has consistently challenged claims that new communication technologies will provide the benefits and limitless choice for audiences in Europe simply because they have the technical capacity to do so. Garnham has argued that fulsome predictions that these new ICTs will 'usher in a new era of cultural freedom, diversity and abundance' concentrate too much on the technical potential of the technologies rather than the social relations that will shape the way their potentials are realised (Garnham 1990: 120).

When considering issues of choice, it is evident that cable and satellite systems have the technical capability to expand the number of channels available and to increase the amount of programming on offer. Extended programme schedules, increased transmission hours and regularly repeated programmes, could also be said to offer increased control and flexibility over when to watch. Developing digital services have the potential to extend this choice further by enabling even more channels (on terrestrial, cable and satellite platforms) and by providing access to a wide range of additional interactive services. In the view of the cable industry, for instance, the constraint on the number of television channels available would much more likely be what the market would bear rather than what technology would allow. However, additional channels do not necessarily provide the diversity of programming and plurality of content which the term choice necessarily implies. Research suggests that promises of a broader range and diversity of programming are not being fulfilled, and in the current socio-economic context, are unlikely to be fulfilled (Blumler and Nossiter 1991; Winston 1998).

Perhaps the first issue to contest is the claim that the advent of new technologies and the deregulation of broadcasting structures would lead to greater competition and thereby offer audiences greater choice and diversity of programming. As the Peacock Report argued, in a market environment audiences' best interests are served by the provision of programming from as many alternative sources of supply as possible. Industry commentators have argued that the opportunities provided by digital technologies mediate against a few providers dominating the market-place. With multiple channels, high quality images and income-generating encryption equipment digital broadcasting ought to provide the opportunity to break BSkyB's 'stranglehold on the new media' (Ferry 1996). Currently, however, BSkyB is the monopoly provider of satellite television in the UK and also accounts for large amounts of the programming provided via cable networks. With its encryption equipment already installed in many homes for existing analogue channels this gives it a head start in the race for digital subscribers. Furthermore, BSkyB are also in the process of consolidating their presence in the German pay-TV market by negotiating with Kirch for a 25 per cent stake in their Premiere World pay-TV business. This investment will be in addition to BSkyB's control of the TM3 channel, which holds the German rights to broadcast Champions League soccer matches, and to their minority stake in Bertelsmann's Vox channel (Boston 1999). The involvement of transnational multimedia corporations such as News Corporation (which owns 40 per cent of BSkyB) has been a growing feature of the deregulated European television sector and BSkyB is just one example of vertical integration where European BSkyB satellite channels are heavily dependent on programming provided by News Corporation's Fox film studios and TV network in the US. This growing concentration of ownership and multimedia synergy reflects both media convergence and the international expansion strategies of the large corporations which reduce competition rather than facilitate it.

Concentration of ownership has significant implications for the range and diversity of programming available to audiences. The UK is second only to the US in the world export of television programming and yet the balance of trade in audio-visual programming between the UK and the US has plummeted from a surplus of £161 million in 1985 to a deficit of £191 million in 1995 (CEC/Tongue 1998). The trend reversed in 1990 and the huge deficit, now £272 million, is largely attributed to BSkyB's reliance on imported American programming and its alleged failure to produce and export original British programming (CEC/ Tongue 1998).[4] UK cable operators also have agreements with US programme providers. The consortium led by Telewest Communications, for example, has agreements with Disney, Universal, MGM and Warner for programme rights. Although this programming undoubtedly includes box-office films, much of it is likely to be cheap, daytime schedule fillers. A programme supply of quality and diversity, offering real choice to the viewer, should include a proportion of original programming produced or commissioned by the programme provider to reflect national cultural traditions (Blumler and Nossiter 1991; Hoffman-Riem 1993). The increasing reliance on US imports reduces the sources and content of programming and does little to reflect national and regional cultures. Furthermore, in the increasingly market-driven broadcasting environment structural concentration of ownership and less accountability may also present conflicts between the range of programming (and opinions) provided and corporate self-interest. News Corporation's withdrawal of the BBC news service from its Star TV network in Asia to promote Chinese business interests has been seen as just such an example of the strength of economic interests. BBC World Service Television, set up in 1991, was reaching in the region of 4 million homes in China, via the Hong Kong based StarTV Network (BBC 1994: 61). When News Corporation bought StarTV in 1993, the BBC service was withdrawn from the network provoking widespread criticism of political pressure and censorship of news bulletins to promote business interests.

Concentration of ownership, however, is only one aspect of the complex contemporary audio-visual industry within which it is evident that economic and commercial pressures play an increasingly important role in determining the range of programming available and hence the scope of choice for audiences. Although a large proportion of revenue for both cable and satellite is increasingly derived from subscription payments and pay-per-view, terrestrial, cable and satellite broadcasters are also heavily dependent on advertising revenues. Speculation by advertising agencies in the late 1980s suggesting that the television advertising markets in most European countries were under-exploited, with opportunity for considerable growth on channels intended for cable and satellite delivery, was arguably a key incentive for investment in these technologies (Lange and Renaud 1989: 162). In addition, opportunities for advertisers on terrestrial broadcast systems opened up by deregulation have added to an increasingly competitive broadcasting environment leading inevitably to financial pressures on programme production and acquisition.

Both the volume of programming required and its cost are influential in determining the choice and quality of material on offer from all television providers. The expansion in the number of television channels and transmission time has meant that the demand for programming since the mid-1980s has risen rapidly and with the current growth of digital transmission is set to increase exponentially. In the rush to fill these schedules the appeal of cheaper imported programming, which in the case of US productions have already recouped costs at home, is far more attractive economically. In the cultural and entertainment industries, the programme production process is both labour and cost intensive. Because of this, there are few productivity gains to be made and relative costs have tended to increase over the years (Baumol and Baumol 1983; Siune and Truetzschler 1992; Garnham and Locksley 1991). The cost of original programming therefore, remains extremely high and economies of scale, as US producers have long understood, are only achieved through reproduction and distribution. As rising costs make original programming produced in the UK and Europe less attractive to cable and satellite channels, US producers have focused programme sales increasingly on Europe as their home film and television markets become saturated. In 1989, Lange and Renaud's research demonstrated that programme rights for a one-hour American drama cost five to ten times less than the cost of a one-hour home produced drama (Lange and Renaud 1989). Current figures indicate that US programming is now likely to cost only ten per cent of programming originating in Europe (CEC 1997b). This is far more profitable in terms of the cost-audience ratio and very attractive to cash-pressed commercial broadcasters.

With the size and growth of the advertising market unreliable, cable and satellite channels have increasingly relied on cheaper ready-made productions rather than investing in more expensive forms of original programming. This reliance on off-the-shelf programming has been intensified by the tendency to raid the archives for old films and popular television series. Some channels, for example, the gameshow channel *Challenge TV*, and *UK Gold*, are composed entirely of this type of material. Digital technologies make the access and reprocessing of this archive material even simpler and can reinforce trends to repackage existing programmes. Recycling, or the endless repetition of a limited range of programmes at regular intervals, is also a method of filling channel schedules, but is usually marketed as providing choice and convenience for audiences (Winston 1998: 319). Downward pressure on budgets also suggests that where new programming is produced, a growing proportion tends to fall within the category of inexpensive quiz shows and lifestyle programming. In general, therefore, rather than access to a wider range and diversity of programming, market forces have contributed to a growing uniformity of television material available to audiences reflecting a marked shift towards entertainment services (Siune and Truetzchler 1992: 95).

Despite these economic pressures, one of the key arguments underpinning the concept of greater choice and access in the market environment is the model of allocative efficiency. This model stresses the ability of the consumer to direct programme providers to supply the right quantity and quality of programming they require at the right price. The economic rationale of commercially funded channels suggests that their need to attract audiences or subscribers ensures that they are more responsive to audience needs and demands. However, the Peacock Report acknowledged that advertising finance tended to prioritise the interests of advertisers rather than audiences. There is little evidence to support the notion that the market environment produces a closer relationship between the audience and the programme provider or that the choice of programming on offer will reflect a broad range of consumer preferences rather than that which the advertisers and broadcasters wish to offer on an economic basis. Increased channel capacity provides the opportunity to stratify audiences to better target advertising or increase subscription, rather than to support narrow, uneconomic market segments.

This assessment does not necessarily imply that audiences are passive or incapable of rational choice but rather that the concept of consumer choice has been actively incorporated into commercial strategies. Recent studies by Ang and others have shown that the notion of an 'active audience' is not necessarily incompatible with a critical assessment of the notion of increased choice provided by new media technologies. It is in some senses 'a sign of heightened cultural contradictions in contemporary society' (Ang 1996: 9). Indeed the concept of an 'active audience' has been well recognised by the television industry itself in terms of the way programming is promoted and audiences targeted. 'This shift in institutional awareness throughout the rapidly globalising media industries, which intensified during the 1980s, signifies the emergence of the 'active audience' at the very heart of corporate concerns' (Ang 1996: 12). The concept of choice has become a means of legitimating the expansion of new media technologies and is a key ingredient in the drive to increase consumption. As Ang argues convincingly, 'the active audience has nothing to do with "resistance", but everything to do with incorporation: the imperative of choice interpellates the audience as "active" ' (Ang 1996: 12).

The changing nature of the broadcasting structures from predominately free-to-air broadcasting services to an increasingly transactional environment based on subscription and pay-per-view inevitably means that equality of access is limited by the audiences' ability to pay for them. In view of the criticism of the actual level of real choice provide by these services, this may not be considered as a significant disadvantage. However, these changes have significant implications for audiences due to their negative impacts on existing free-to-air broadcasting services, the restrictions they impose on access to a whole range of programming previously available without charge, and the implications they pose for access to additional services which will ultimately be delivered alongside digital television.

In terms of revenue, competition for advertising impacts on the commercial viability and programme quality of existing broadcasting channels. As early as 1992, the cable relay of UK and other English language channels in Eire was recognised as a key factor in diverting revenue away from the public service broadcaster (financed by licence fee and advertising income), resulting in cutbacks in services and programming (Euromedia Research Group 1992: 109–11). In addition, increased competition for audience ratings, which is vital for attracting advertising revenue, influences the programming patterns of existing broadcasters. In the increasingly competitive environment, if national broadcasters and cable and satellite channels are competing for the same audiences, as well as sources of finance, there is a tendency for national channels to compete at the same level and produce the same type of programming. This so-called 'dumbing-down' process has been identified in contemporary reports of declining television standards and has been referred to as the *Dallasification of culture* in academic accounts (Collins 1990; Siune and Truetzschler 1992). Even where the availability of cable and satellite channels does not appear to have affected the proportion of serious and popular programming on existing channels, research has shown that prime-time viewing has been increasingly filled with entertainment programmes, with more serious material relegated to less popular hours (Euromedia Research Group 1992: 27). This is a pattern increasingly recognisable in the television schedules of UK terrestrial broadcasters, reflected, to some extent, by the move in March 1999 of the ITV flagship *News At Ten* to a later 11pm slot. ITV have argued that this gives them greater flexibility to schedule quality dramas, documentaries and films in peak-time but industry analysts have suggested that the move reflects the intensifying battle for audiences and ratings, and that 'the only justification for the move was to clear the way for popular programming' (Horsman quoted in *Evening Standard* 12 May 1999).[5] Curran has argued that, with few rules imposed on new cable and satellite channel providers to ensure a balance of programming, 'the new stations turned, like their American counterparts, to the lowest denominator of pop, chat, soap and sport' (Curran and Seaton 1997: 204). Where the diversity and range of programming available on existing networks is undermined by competition with these cable and satellite channels, there is a tendency to reduce choice rather than enhance it.

Another significant concern is the increasing migration of certain areas of programming away from free-to-air television providers to subscription and pay-per-view systems. Whilst it has been noted that encryption technology and the set-top box enable consumers to express their programming preferences more directly to channel providers, it is also the means by which access is restricted only to consumers who have subscribed to specific packages or individual pay-per-view events. As the introduction to this chapter indicates, some popular programming, such as national and international sports, film and other events, have been identified by BSkyB as the most successful way of building subscription and pay-per-view audiences. They have become the so-called 'killer applications' for which the Internet is still searching and which will drive audience take-up of new digital television services. These strategies increasingly escalate the cost of popular programming which, in the case of sport, is clearly linked to the social and cultural traditions of British audiences. The question of ownership of these broadcast rights, and the way they are utilised to reserve access exclusively to users who are able to pay, presents a growing problem of inequality of access. The ITAP report in 1982, despite its overwhelming support for cable development, acknowledged that some people would be adversely affected by the new media and recognised that 'the loss of major sporting events to cable was the principal concern...measures would have to be taken to prevent this happening' (Hollins 1984:59). Yet, when the rights for live coverage of Premier League football matches came up for renegotiation in 1992, BSkyB's bid of £304 million was accepted in a deal which allowed exclusive coverage of sixty live matches per season on Sky Sports and provided the BBC with recorded highlights on Saturday nights (Chippindale and Franks 1991: 323). Other broadcasters were unable to match the bid based on advertising or licence fee revenue alone. The strength of BSkyB's bid was underpinned by the need to drive dish sales and the expected level of income to be derived from subscription. The government rejected calls for a full enquiry, refusing to intervene in what they considered commercial negotiations.[6] In 1996, BSkyB secured the rights for a further four years for £670 million (Independent Television Commission 1998) and have used them as the focal point of their drive for new digital subscribers and pay-per-view events.[7] ONdigital, the digital terrestrial television provider, has also secured a deal with ITV which means that audiences will have to subscribe to the digital service to see half of the European Champions League matches from September 1999 (Cleveland-Peck and Hammersley 1999).

The implications of these developments are clear when it is noted that, for example, live coverage of Premier League matches is now restricted to Sky Sports subscribers who, in the year ending 31 December 1998, made up only an estimated 1.6 per cent of the total television audience share (Independent Television Commission 1999)[8]. A similar pattern is reflected elsewhere in Europe with key matches in Italy and Spain available only to minority audiences via pay-per-view and subscription channels (Hughes 1999). Although sporting events are currently the key focus of concern in the debate over this siphoning-off of key areas of programming the issues of exclusion and inequality of access apply across the television spectrum. Many popular entertainment programmes, which have built a strong audience on free-to-air channels, have subsequently been bought up by satellite channels. With the audience seen increasingly as a consumer in the transactional environment, private access for private gain is rapidly replacing the system of public access for the public good.

Digital television services are also now poised to offer a whole range of communication products and services in parallel with broadcasting. Television has several years advance on the Internet as a medium for delivering broadcast quality programming as well as providing a user-friendly interface with audiences. It offers a gateway to these new services which audiences will find familiar and accessible. Yet conditional access systems and subscription costs makes it likely that the ability to receive them will be restricted by income in the same way as the broadcast services they accompany.

THE FUTURE OF BROADCASTING: PAY-PER-VIEW?

This chapter has argued against the claim that recent technological and organisational changes in the broadcasting environment have fulfilled expectations of providing greater choice and access for audiences. Contrary to the rhetoric, new technologies of cable and satellite distribution have not opened the television market-place to new and diverse sources of programming but, rather, have resulted in even greater concentration and cross-media owership. Economic imperatives have limited the range of real choice for viewers on new satellite and cable channels whilst, at the same time, the increased competition for audiences and revenue has had negative impacts on the services provided by existing free-to-air broadcasters. The growing transactional nature of the audience-programme provider relationship, and the increase in subscription and pay-per-view services, has resulted in exclusion rather than greater access in some areas. These trends are likely to accelerate as new competing digital systems play a more prominent role in the television sector. The market-led environment is unlikely to provide equality of access to a wide range of quality programming unless more positive programming obligations are imposed on commercial providers to ensure their schedules include more original programming from the UK. One possible way of encouraging this would be the example of the obligation imposed by the French government on their pay-TV channel, *Canal Plus*, to invest 12 per cent of its annual turnover in French and European programming (CEC/Tongue 1998: 2). This model could be applied to satellite and cable television providers licensed in the UK and would have benefits both for increasing the plurality of programming available to UK audiences and for widening opportunities for domestic programme producers. The structure of the market inevitably means that satellite and digital providers, eager to expand their subscriber bases, target the types of programming which have already developed a proven appeal on existing free-to-air channels. In sport, this has progressively led to the two-tier market structure, predicted by Garnham in the 1980s (1990: 125), with choice becoming increasingly expensive and the sports schedules of existing broadcasters increasingly impoverished and devoid of national sports events. The question of broadcasting rights, therefore, also needs to be reviewed to ensure that their exclusivity does not determine access solely on the grounds of ability to pay. Finally, this chapter has argued that, despite the acknowledged limitations of public service broadcasting, its commitment to the social, cultural and political needs of its audience rather than the economic imperatives of the market, presents a powerful argument for its continuing importance in the future digital environment. The existing public service broadcasting services in the UK need continued support to ensure that those unable to subscribe to additional services still have access to a range of diverse, high quality information and entertainment.

NOTES

1 Richard Keys, Sky Sports anchorman quoted in Cleveland-Peck and Hammersley 1999.
2 The Protocol to the Amsterdam Treaty dated June 1997 on public service broadcasting recognises that 'the system of public service broadcasting in the Member States is directly related to the democratic, social and cultural needs of each society and to the need to preserve media pluralism' (CEC 1997a).
3 A limited pay-cable experiment was piloted in 1980 with thirteen schemes licensed for a period of two years to ascertain whether pay-television could develop side-by-side with variable community channels. The trial met with only limited success and the focus of debate shifted to political discussion of the wider industrial and economic potentials of cable development (Hollins 1984).
4 Cable and satellite channels, mainly BSkyB, have claimed that when they tried to buy programming from the BBC and ITV they were turned away (Hayes 1999).
5 It is interesting to note that in the first two months after the schedule change audience ratings were often down on the regular six million viewers who tuned in to *News At Ten*, reflecting, at least initially, some dissatisfaction with the standard of programmes in its place (Hosking 1999).

6 ITV, whose bid for the rights was rejected, subsequently appealed to the High Court but failed to win their case (ITC 1998).
7 An estimated 20,000 BSkyB subscribers paid £7.95 to watch the first live pay-per-view league football match between Oxford United and Sunderland on 28 February 1999 (Cleveland-Peck and Hammersley 1999).
8 Total combined audience share of three Sky Sports channels, Independent Television Commission, January 1999.

5

LIMITED HORIZONS (INC.)

Access, democracy and technology in community television in Canada

Herbert F. Pimlott

When community access television[1] was launched more than twenty years ago, it set imaginations afire with its utopian promises: ordinary people communicating directly with one another and with government, reversing the traditional top-down command model of both communications and government. It was the convergence of technology and demands for social change which launched community access TV as a viable, democratic alternative to the older hierarchical, authoritarian forms of government and communications: interest turned from the 'global village' to 'electronic town hall democracy' (Dolan 1984). However, as with the promise of every new media technology this century, community access TV also promised to democratise the process of government through citizen participation in direct communication with the powerful, vested interests in society. Somewhat paradoxically, it was a Canadian government agency which initiated the process, institutionalising access from the top down, while in the US, a more complex and contradictory development took place which included grassroots organising.

This chapter examines the relationship between technology and inequality by investigating the attempts by the community access TV movement during the 1960s, 1970s and 1980s in Canada and the US to redress the imbalance between citizens and the government. The purpose was to provide access to new communication technology (video, cable) and the requisite technical skills so that ordinary citizens would be able to 'have their say', which in turn would stimulate and re-energise the apathetic and unmotivated to become involved in the democratic process. Underlying this belief is the assumption that democracy is strengthened when people participate in the processes of communication and governance: the greater the participation in communication the more likely that ordinary people will benefit. After examining some of the key concepts underlying discussions about community television, such as the liberal-democratic theory of the media, the information society, access and the public sphere, this chapter offers an assessment of the trajectory of community access TV in Canada which will provide an understanding of some of the problems facing community access TV and the limitations of the technologically determinist claims made on its behalf. This chapter provides an historical parallel to consider similar claims made on behalf of the Internet.

PROMISES, PROMISES: THE 'INFORMATION SOCIETY' AND ACCESS

One of the problems with the debates concerning the 'information society' and whether or not we are living in a 'information age' or in the midst of a 'technological revolution', is the way the issue has been conceptualised, especially in relation to inequality in society. The increasing divisions of inequality in contemporary global capitalism at all levels (national, regional, local or global) have been re-classified. We have moved from the social and economic inequalities of the workplace, office and factory floor, where inequality or 'difference' was between those who sold their labour and those who bought it, that is, inequalities between workers and capitalists, to the inequalities of the 'information age' and the 'post-industrial society' with 'information-haves' and 'information-have-nots'. This is a rather 'neat-and-tidy' way of dismissing a wide range of inequities that can be treated as a 'lack', not of money or resources, but of education. Even the lack of information is seen more of a case of education providing the solution to a problem which is economically, and hence socially and politically, structured and effected by active agencies. The problem is that it is based upon a rather static and passive conception of human beings and of 'information' as something which can simply be equated to more 'real' commodities such as shoes or bread. Such a conceptualisation suggests that to fix the problem it is simply necessary to redistribute some of the commodities from the haves to the have-nots. Problems begin to arise because information is not a simple commodity: once information has been produced as a commodity, the costs of reproduction approach zero. However, the production and consumption of information relies on the ability of people to manipulate information, which in turn requires the relevant skills, knowledge, and 'know-how'.

The rise of the mass media during the late nineteenth and early twentieth centuries led to the elite's fears of 'anarchy' and the 'masses', which were euphemisms for the rise of democratic rule through the extension of universal suffrage to ordinary people, including women and the 'property-less'. With the rise of mass societies, the ability of ordinary people to have any control over their day-to-day existence, however, continued to be circumscribed by the remoteness of government, the state and big business. The press became increasingly important, acting as a substitute for the people in keeping watch over the actions of those in authority. This role has changed during the twentieth century with the increasing profitability and importance of the cultural industries to global media conglomerates, which have become powerful bodies in their own right, often seeking the freedom to do as they choose, regardless of national governments; yet they remain accountable to no-one but their owners and shareholders and, therefore, the global media represent a much greater threat to democracy than most governments.

Traditionally, concerns over 'access' have been articulated in a similar way by information society theorists. The media are taken as given and debates over access tend to be overwhelmingly concerned with the economic or technological: people's access is only discussed in terms of whether they can afford to purchase TV sets or programmes (such as satellite, cable, pay-per-view), pay for TV licences (as in the UK) and/or receive the signals transmitted via satellites or cable.[2] However, the understanding of access must be broadened and used in a way which incorporates and addresses audiences as citizens and which argues that the limitations to access as a concept have been overwhelmingly pre-determined by trans-national corporations and the state (e.g. regulatory and policy frameworks). Thus, drawing upon those theorists such as

Brecht (1930), Benjamin (1969) and Enzensberger (1976), who have pointed out that new communication and media technologies have liberating possibilities and can be used in ways which invert or subvert the traditional capitalist and state-authoritarian models of top-down control, I argue from a position which supports the idea that problems with both modern media and government are really about the social organisation and control of the technology rather than the technology itself. I argue that the problems with democracy stem from the continuation of capitalist organisation and control of communication and the market imperative, which only benefits those who already have sufficient capital to purchase a newspaper or television station, and limits democracy by restricting participation in the public sphere (in terms, for example, of debates, agenda-setting, etc.).[3] It is not only participation in elections or consuming information but having the opportunity and possibility to communicate to others that is vital to the life-blood of any democracy.

This chapter, therefore, is underpinned by the assumption that the greater the numbers of ordinary people participating in public communication, the more it develops and strengthens the democratic process. Access to technology, including both know-how and machinery, is a positive development which will deepen and extend democracy. Implicitly, if not explicitly, special interest groups (media corporations, cable companies, TV stations) will oppose any such undertaking if they are not able to profit directly from it. In Canada, community access TV was actually instituted top-down by the federal government, acting in response to demands from below.

The community access TV movement in north America generally is interesting because not only does it enable us to explore these issues and their consequences, it also offers a chance to reflect upon the current debates and claims being made for the Internet and other electronic media. Community access TV and the Internet were both introduced with the rhetoric of greater democracy for, and input from, ordinary citizens. Much has been made of the Internet's promise for revolutionising how we are governed, instituting democratic controls over the state and enabling ongoing electronic referenda on every issue from traffic planning to international trade; yet there is little or no acknowledgement of the realities behind the introduction of such new technology. It is arguable that there is a closer fit between Internet rhetoric (or more accurately, hyperbole) and the assumptions that the (so-called) 'free market' will deliver democracy, but clearly the promotional rhetorics surrounding both community access TV and Internet technologies are 'technologically determinist'. As this chapter will show, the situation of community access TV is quite different from the utopian claims often made for new media technologies: the technology by itself does not determine its impact so much as the social, economic, political and cultural factors that shape how new technologies are employed. The experience of community access TV demonstrates the chasm between the democratic promises of a new technology heralded to the public and the realities upon which such promises foundered. Before going on to examine the experience of community access TV in Canada, it is necessary to consider both the dominant liberal-democratic theory of the media and the theory of the public sphere, in order to re-think the process of communication and participation in a democracy.

THE MARKETPLACE OF IDEAS

In liberal-democratic theory, media are integral to the democratic process, acting as the 'marketplace of ideas'. Legal guarantees of individual rights of free speech, free assembly and association, and freedom to publish (or broadcast) are not just the cornerstones of democracy, but constitute its very foundations. This means that anyone can publish or broadcast their ideas, but it is only insofar as they are able to reach enough people who can be persuaded to purchase their media output, that they will be able to realise any such hope. While liberal-democratic theory believes that 'the truth will out', the marketplace (and the competitors involved, particularly global media moguls) actually act in ways which censor, limit or even obliterate messages and meanings. Thus the marketplace becomes the arbiter of ideas and therefore the media that most closely 'reflect' or 'represent' the public's opinions become 'popular': these preferences are determined by sales figures for newspapers and periodicals or audience ratings for radio and television. Hence the views of some journalists who argue that unlike parliamentary politicians who only have to face the electorate every four or five years, newspapers are subject to the equivalent of an election every day they go on sale. The marketplace model of the free exchange of ideas is based upon an unspoken utopian ideal of a 'level playing field', where all ideas are able to compete equally, and it simply equates purchase of a particular newspaper (or the viewing of a programme) with agreement with its political views or message, ignoring other possible factors which affect the take-up of newspapers.[4]

However, it is clear that this simplistic understanding about the relationship between the media and ideas does not actually work in practice. For example, the sales and audience ratings for different media may reflect a very limited choice of ideas which the public ends up being constrained to read, listen to or watch. Liberal-democratic theorists would counter that such people could just as easily not purchase the newspapers or magazines, available. But how does such a choice register in the marketplace of ideas? The only alternative on offer for those whose voices are excluded is to establish their own newspapers, radio or TV stations, which is beyond the reach of the overwhelming mass of people because of the prohibitive financial costs and regulatory structures. Thus the market ensures that what counts is money rather than ideas or principles (of, for example, equality, liberty, free speech) and confirms that only the wealthiest will be able to ensure their views are heard.

Since the difficulties arise because of the costs, monopoly control (in, for example, cable provision) or scarcity (in, for example, broadcasting frequencies), the logical outcome of such a situation would be to enforce access for others to the media which already exist: ensuring the freedom for all to publicise or broadcast their views through existing media is one way to redress the imbalance in the marketplace of ideas. This is more likely to produce a real sense of representation of differing viewpoints within any single newspaper, radio or TV station. If every medium gave over a portion of its space or programming to the ordinary public, it would also mean that no one outlet would be forced to cope with representing all marginalised groups, which is the way in which access channels are expected to operate.

One other point to consider about liberal-democratic theory is that of the news media's self-appointed role as a 'public watchdog', exposing abuses of power and privilege. This is intimately tied up with the notion of the press as the 'fourth estate' (after church, nobility and the commoners) which has a duty to keep corruption and the potential usurpation of democracy by others in check. Again, a problem has arisen because the media themselves have substantial vested interests with their own special privileges which they seek to protect and, as many commercial organisations become more powerful than most countries in the world, the potential abuse of power comes not only from the state, government and the political class, but also from powerful, publicly-unaccountable organisations like transnational corporations and especially media conglomerates and moguls because of their potential to influence people's beliefs. However, because conservatives and liberals interpret this as restricting state power only, the applicability of this theory is limited.

THE PUBLIC SPHERE AND COMMUNITY ACCESS TELEVISION

A different approach which enables the application of a normative standard against which to judge the contribution and effectivity of different media to democracy is that of the public sphere, as elaborated by Jürgen Habermas. Habermas developed the theory of the public sphere by drawing upon a historical analysis of its development in Britain, France and Germany from the seventeenth to the early twentieth centuries. The public sphere is an institution which comes into being whenever private individuals gather together, outside of any state or economic activity, to engage in rational-critical debate (Habermas 1974: 51). Through the public sphere, citizens restrict power through formal (elections, referenda) and informal (polls, demonstrations) means, ensuring that neither government nor private organisations exceed their authority.

The media play an important role in making public the general interests of private individuals, as long as they permit open access to free rational-critical debate (critical publicity). However, once individual rights of private economic competition were established, the press lost interest in furthering civil rights. In mass society, not only do the media 'facilitate' the public sphere (albeit in limited ways), they often *become* the public sphere (or 'simulate' it). Private control of the media limits the individual's influence in the public sphere because there is no guarantee of democratic process or accountability in private organisations, except within co-operatives and unions which maintain their own internal public sphere, though these may differ in terms of democratic process and accountability.

Public participation in the governing of society is limited to 'acclamatory' forms, such as choosing politician A or B, instead of putting forward their own choices or representing themselves. Since the media can promote, defuse or block private and public interests and opinions, the formation of public opinion has to be secured by a legal guarantee. But the effectiveness of the public sphere depends upon individual rights being interpreted as guarantees of participation. Thus the degree of a society's democratisation can be measured by the extent to which critical publicity prevails over 'staged publicity'. Critical publicity relies upon access to the public sphere, guaranteed by law. It is not just the right to free assembly and free speech but access to the means *to publicise* one's thoughts and the right *to communicate* to other members of the polity.

However, the public sphere is no longer made up of 'a plurality of equally empowered and competing parts', if it ever was (Hohendahl 1979: 108; see also the collection in Calhoun 1992). Reflecting class structures, the powerful and the wealthy are at the top of the collective public sphere, while marginal interests are part of the counter-public sphere at the bottom (Negt 1978: 65ff).[5] However, if the counter-public sphere is separated from the collective public sphere, it ceases to have any influence; access should mean marginal private interests being made public through the mass broadcasting system, not ghettoising them (Salter 1988: 238). Nevertheless, the concept of the public sphere is useful as a normative means for thinking through the democratic potential, claims and rationale of any public medium.[6]

Crucial to the bourgeois public sphere, according to Habermas, was a public that critically debated culture. Today, however, as the commodification of culture has contributed to its public consumption, there is less of an engagement with rational-critical dialogue, and the 'active audience' theory notwithstanding, public discourse lacks a sense of engagement with all citizens.[7] Community access TV proponents have put the emphasis on the community channel as a medium for citizens to *process* their experiences rather than as a means of *publicising* different opinions (that is, acting as a mechanism for distributing different viewpoints), an emphasis which is a direct result of its origins (see below). As the mass media expanded access to the public sphere by commercialising participation in it, the expanded public sphere 'lost its political character'(e.g. the rise of 'infotainment') (Habermas 1989: 169).

Technologically determinist promises of a new era of 'participatory democracy' are quickly forgotten once the new technology becomes established as part of the infrastructure. It does not presuppose that the Internet or other new technologies might not actually have the capacity to realise the political benefits for which its proponents make claims, but that which will effectively shape the Internet and other new technologies will be the 'vested interests' (business organisations, media conglomerates, the state, etc.), whose *raison d'être* is primarily, if not solely, to maximise profits. Indeed, the introduction of community access TV also has to recognise the fortuitous circumstances by which social and political events of the 1960s helped to bring about partial successes: without the rise of social and community activism, community access TV might have been much more limited from the start than it actually became.[8]

Community access television should be seen as an update of Brecht's 1930 vision of radio's potential, in spite of its economic, social and institutional limitations (Brecht 1930). Walter Benjamin's writings about the potential of new media technology have been taken up more readily than those of Brecht, even though Benjamin also had expressed concerns over technology's limitations (Benjamin 1969). Nevertheless, the convergence of technology and demands for social change launched community TV as a viable democratic concept: the 'global village' turned into an 'electronic town hall democracy' (Dolan 1984). It established the idea of community TV as a tool for social change in the public's imagination. Social change could come about in the *process* of communication. The media would be the means by which any community could exert influence over its own destiny. Community activists believed that the power of technology would enable Canadians to communicate freely and to realise progressive social and political change. At its best, community TV has helped communities to realise their own solutions through public discussion, while at its worst it reproduces the existing power relations in society. With more than 300 channels across Canada, community TV is still the most accessible 'public forum', because access is guaranteed by law. Yet audiences remain small, and community access TV fails to elicit much interest, even among social and community activists, although this was not always the case.

This lack of interest is partly reflected in the dearth of written material outside the US literature on the subject between the mid-1970s and the mid-1990s.[9] Most writing on community television concentrates on the early years of its 'utopian promise.' Laws guaranteed access for all, and yet there is a sense that community TV was not as accessible as the managers made out. Dissenting voices could be heard at public hearings. However, differences in access structures, programming and ownership had a greater effect on its ability to function as a democratic medium.

BEGINNINGS: VIDEO FOR SOCIAL CHANGE

The inspiration for community television in north America grew out of the Canadian National Film Board's (NFB) Challenge For Change/Société Nouvelle (CFC) projects during the 1960s. These projects reflected the NFB's committed social documentary approach. The most famous project, on Fogo Island, near Newfoundland, on Canada's Atlantic coast, established the idea of community television in the public imagination. With their main source of income, fishing, in decline, unemployment at sixty percent, and divided by religious and ancestral bigotry, the Fogo Islanders had little hope of overcoming their differences and had become resigned to the federal government's plans to relocate them away from their island. However, CFC film-makers who went to the island were determined not to repeat the mistakes of the first CFC project in Montreal, where a fly-on-the-wall documentary of welfare families exposed the film's participants to the ridicule of their neighbours after it was broadcast. They were helped in this matter by the new porta-pak cameras and recorders.

The porta-pak video technology was perfect for the situation faced by the CFC film-makers on Fogo Island. The portability of the new technology meant that it was much easier to carry the video cameras from village to village around the island (in these days of the single-hand held 'palmcorder', it is easy to forget that camera equipment was much heavier only thirty-odd years ago.) Crucially, unlike the case of film, there was no need to send the footage far away to a processing centre in one of the large cities, so the shots could be discussed right there and then by participants, community and film-makers. The third most noted element was the immediate play-back capabilities of video technology which enabled participants to have immediate feedback into, and control over, how they were represented on screen. Both participants and professionals could examine all recording as soon as it had taken place and re-shoot whatever they were unhappy with (the costs were also reduced because any unwanted video tape could be re-used for other shots).

The immediacy of video also contributed to its use as a tool for 'animating' community discussions: when filming in one village reached completion, the CFC film-makers moved on to the next, where the other villagers were able to comment on the similarity of problems and issues facing their neighbours. As the filming progressed, Fogo Islanders overcame their own prejudices towards one another and were able to work together on common solutions to common problems: this co-operation was a direct result of the film-making *process*, rather than the product. The Canadian federal government was compelled to shelve its re-location plans for the islanders as the latter became organised; the government responded to the islanders' new initiatives and self-organisation by helping them launch a fishing co-operative and marketing board.

The Fogo Island project's success had a ripple effect, helping to inspire the idea of community television throughout north America.[10] It demonstrated how the media could play a positive role in social change and provide the means by which people in any community could help re-establish a degree of control over their own destiny. At a time when demands for social change were widespread, the technological development of the new media (cable, porta-pak video) seemed to offer the means to overcome government aloofness; if the people could voice their opinions, then surely those in power would have to listen.

However, one crucial aspect of the CFC Fogo Island project had been overlooked. While the technology's playback capability had enabled participants and film-makers to discuss different shots, it was not the porta-pak which decided how it would be used. That decision was a very conscious one taken by the film-makers themselves to give the subjects of their documentary greater control. The film-makers refused to use any shot without the consent of the subjects, who also represented themselves on camera in true *verité* documentary style. Thus, the film-makers remained in control even if they chose to give up that power to the participants. In the heat of the moment, the role of the CFC professional film-makers themselves was overlooked in favour of what the new technology could offer.

CABLE ACCESS TELEVISION: PRIVATE INDUSTRY OR PUBLIC UTILITY?

During the early years of access TV, when the cable operators were less knowledgeable about what the community channel should do and be, they ended up leaving it to local activists. This meant that the commitment to local community access television was motivated by desires for social and political change rather than as a means of training for a career. As community activists became involved in making access TV, local vested interests (e.g. political and business figures) became less than enthusiastic, especially when their own activities were scrutinised or criticised. One of the earliest and most renowned example occurred in Port Arthur,[11] Ontario, in 1971, when a community cable talk show, 'Town Talk', which was critical of the local government, was shut down by the cable operator despite its popularity (which clearly flies in the face of the claims made by liberal-democratic theorists and proponents of the 'marketplace of ideas'). Thus, even in its infancy, community access TV events revealed that community channel programming decisions were not going to be left to the community. Possible redress appears to be limited since the government regulatory body was less than enthusiastic about intervening against the monopolies that control access and facilities.[12]

Established in 1968, at virtually the same time that community television was born, the Canadian Radio-television and Telecommunications Commission (CRTC) had the means to secure an active, open-access forum by providing guidelines and enforcing regulations. It had the power to issue and revoke licences, to act on complaints, to permit rate increases or not. It was even proposed that the promises made by applicants 'should be made contractual conditions of licences, enforceable by prosecution or suspension of the licences' (Hardin 1985: 13). Yet the CRTC appears unwilling to revoke licences, except in the most flagrant cases of abuse.[13] In 1990, for example, despite four dissenting opinions, the CRTC approved Rogers Cablesystems' take-over of more cable licences in Greater Vancouver, increasing its ownership of cable to 76 per cent of all households in the region (CRTC 1989–90).[14]

Cable's near universality in Canada and the manner of its monopoly provision[15] make it effectively a 'public utility'; government regulation is necessary, therefore, to prevent unjustified rate increases or any other abuse. In exchange for their monopolies, the CRTC requires cable operators to provide the public with the training, equipment and resources to 'cablecast' their concerns via community channels, although even this is funded out of the subscriptions paid by the public. The CRTC did require cable operators to provide the minimum resources for a community access channel at first. In its 1975 policy statement on community TV, the primary social commitment of the cable licensee was supposed to be to the community channel. Gradually, though, the CRTC has permitted the cable industry more control over the channel, while retreating from the enforcement of regulations in overseeing the guidelines (Layng et al 1989; Blaine 1983). This became more obvious in the 1980s.

In 1986, as part of its review of Canada's broadcasting system, the Caplan-Sauvageau Task Force recognised the necessity to split cable licences into two: one for the cable companies, who would supply the signals to the public as before; and the other for the community channel, to be controlled by elected community boards. The cable industry would turn over the ten percent of their revenues earmarked for community TV to these boards. The cable companies were 'outraged', claimed they felt 'insulted' and attacked the task force members for being out of touch with the 'reality' of community TV (Goldberg 1990; McNulty 1988).

The experience in Québec, however, with the Association of Community Communication Councils of Québec (ROCCQ)[16] was a good example of how to involve the community through advisory boards to oversee the community channel. Nevertheless, the CRTC refused to recognise them because it was concerned that any recognition of ROCCQ would mean that the federal government would lose jurisdiction over cable communications: it claimed that such matters were national and not provincial concerns. However, the Québec provincial government funded ROCCQ anyway, providing extra funding for the community channels, which even enabled the community channels to mount news programming. However, during the 1980s the ROCCQ's situation changed for the worst as the Québec government cut its funding and the cable companies refused to let ROCCQ have control over community TV resources. Throughout Canada, the CRTC has rejected almost every application from community coalitions or co-operatives, regardless of the degree of public support for these projects or their viability (Hardin 1985).[17]

The closeness between the CRTC and the cable industry has to do with other battles, particularly as the cable industry became an ally of the CRTC in its regulatory battles over the airwaves with the broadcasting industry. The CRTC used cable as a lever over the broadcasters (see Salter 1988). Cable is big business with average revenues of one billion dollars a year. A few leading Canadian cable outfits have international interests,[18] while the industry produces approximately 7,000 hours of community programming a month.[19] The Canadian Cable Television Association (CCTA), the cable industry's lobby group, runs awards ceremonies for different types of programming every year and while these awards may provide encouragement to staff and volunteers to produce good programming, they also serve to encourage conformity to professional standards, which may or may not be a good thing. (The difference relates to whether it is more important to ensure conformity to broadcast standards, in which the role of professionals becomes dominant, or whether it is more important to encourage participation and community access TV to develop its own particular aesthetics, with or without the assistance of professionals.)

During the 1970s, the CRTC carried out two community channel surveys. These pointed to a significant decline in the amount of programming produced solely by community members: from 78 per cent of programmes in 1972 to 44 per cent in 1978. One factor in this rapid decline may be a growing disenchantment with the corporations' bureaucratic control, as well as the cable operators' increasing unwillingness to leave the community channel to chance. The third, most recent, survey conducted in 1988 states that it is archaic to differentiate between 'locally-originated' (staff-initiated) programming and 'access' (volunteer-initiated) programming, as 'a mix of volunteers and cable staff are involved in most programming' (Layng et al 1989: 22). This statement, taken in conjunction with the development of the community channel's bureaucratic structures, stress on high production standards, increasing sophistication of technology (and the consequent reliance on professionals for advice) and imitation of broadcasting aesthetics means that the figure has, at the very least, not increased, and realistically, if anything, it has probably decreased.

COMMUNITY ACCESS TELEVISION: PRODUCT OR POLITICS?

Community television was an attempt to meet public demands for access to the public sphere through the new media on the one hand, and on the other to satisfy the demands of a rapidly growing industry seeking private gain in areas under public authority. This is the conflict between the private sphere (economic interests) and the public sphere (political interests). The privatisation of access to the public sphere continues as media ownership is concentrated into even fewer private hands. Hence the CRTC guarantees a legal right of access: no-one should be refused the right to use the community channel, except for reasons of libel, slander or obscenity. But accessibility means letting the public control the production and access structures as much as the content. The marginal status of community television limits its role as a public sphere. The audience reach is restricted by a lack of publicity and public awareness. The community channel has a crucial role in legitimising local issues and people; by having local issues, groups and individuals on television, it can help make these interests more legitimate in the eyes of the public.

Community access television in Canada was meant to be about enabling the grassroots to speak, to voice their concerns. Yet it has been instituted top down, with the government responding to public demands of the time. Rather than turning the 'cablewaves' over to the citizens, the government gave organised private interests (corporations) control. This mixing of private and public power (Habermas's concept of 'refeudalisation') means private interests have the rights over 'public property'(airwaves). Legal responsibility rests with the private interests who have a relatively free hand in its operation, subject only to government recall of the licence. Moreover the state's reluctance to revoke licence increases as time passes further diminishes the public's right of recourse. Private interests act as gatekeepers: as they are legally responsible for content, they will use *their* right to censor programmes and discourage participation. The identification of the community channel with the private cable operator propagates this idea. People are unlikely to demand access if they cannot identify with the channel. Another problem arises from the fact that those private interests that are responsible for what goes on air are also responsible for 'animating' (motivating) the community to participate.

For the public sphere to be effective, it will be necessary to introduce it into private organisations. Large corporations are less susceptible to public pressure than small, co-operative or non-profit operators because they are outside public scrutiny, since most of them sit outside the jurisdiction of local, regional and even national governments. However, even if there were a public sphere inside a private organisation, it does not necessarily mean people will exercise their rights. It is partly the structures of power that deprive people of the ability and willpower to take control over their lives; a fact which was revealed by the extent to which individuals and organisations were employed to 'animate' participants in community access TV. This was the contradiction within the community TV movement during the 1970s, when community 'animators' were hired in order to get the community out to use the channel, which ostensibly had come about in the first place due to public pressure to speak for and represent themselves. A bureaucratic access structure has arisen in place of autonomous organisation and control. The nature of such structures serves to discourage people, especially those who hold marginal views.

The logic of copying broadcast television aesthetics and conventions only makes sense if community TV is competing for the same audiences and advertisers. By differentiating itself, the community channel could create a space for the public sphere, especially at a time when the proliferation of channels threatens to overwhelm both the community channel and its role as a public sphere. The public sphere is not limited to those who speak, but includes those who listen (audiences). It is important that groups actively work to build audiences as the media access group, Metro Media, did. Based in Vancouver during the 1970s, Metro Media helped social and community organisations produce, distribute and broadcast videos (Goldberg 1990; Tuer 1994). Unlike many of its contemporary video producers, Metro Media created a dynamic, albeit small, counter-public sphere not only by providing access to participants but also by promoting their videos to the public in order to build an audience.

Censorship is at the operator's discretion. Recourse in such matters is more limited since private interests are not as accountable as public bodies and some companies openly refuse to cablecast programmes. One argument put forward by cable operators for their right to censor, refuse or edit programming is that the community is not responsible enough to oversee the community channel. However, this sensibility about a community's responsibility is tempered when it might entail extra costs. For example, Rogers Cablesystems has argued against having to introduce a six second telephone delay mechanism to screen obscene comments because of the responsible nature of community participants: it would cost $80,000 for each community channel, a very expensive proposition for any corporation with lots of community channels (Ackroyd in Burnaby Community TV 1992; Carver 1992). Outright censorship does not have to be used, since caution itself is not very conducive to producing controversial programming – a likely outcome of marginal views – even though that was the rationale for which the community channel was established in the first place (see Spiller's submission to the CRTC 1990).

CONCLUSION

The difference between community TV today and thirty years ago lies in the different emphases in production: product versus process. Thirty years ago the focus was on the importance of learning by doing and producing for special audiences rather than trying to appeal to everybody. The value of a video produced in the process approach is limited outside its immediate locale, subject matter and participants. The professionalisation of community programming has led to the present emphasis on the product, and this emphasis is based upon technical expertise in meeting broadcast aesthetics and conventions, in terms of appealing to a wider audience.[20] The specificity of the particular place

> has to be diluted in order for it to transcend the bounda-
> ries of place, culture and class – which, paradoxically,
> means that the original process that engendered the video
> recedes into the background. Yet it is this *original* process,
> this experience of democracy, that the video is trying to
> communicate as being not only fundamental but necessary
> for change.
>
> (Burnett 1991: 59)

It is in this process of producing the video that the participants constitute the public sphere. Skills become an important part of ensuring that those who are normally denied access will not have to continue relying on animators or professionals to provide them with the technical know-how, which provides a form of mediated access, and such access is not necessarily liberating as technical decisions can often mask political decisions.

The influence of the cable 'community network' concept works both for and against community input. The cable network, like any broadcast network, can broadcast the same programming to several stations at once, which can mean less available time for local programming. On the other hand, community programming thought to be of wider appeal could be broadcast to all, which could mean exposure for important issues. It can also mean that the topicality of local issues are replaced by programmes with universal appeal. Each station receiving the same programming can reduce the amount of funding for community TV.

Community television's main strength lies in its coverage of local politics. It can have a complementary effect because broadcasting related to local elections raises the profile of community issues while at the same time potentially increasing the community's interest in a channel, even if only temporarily. Undoubtedly, community TV's coverage has been more successful than that of broadcast television because the channels deal with local issues in depth. Live coverage of council meetings is a cheap way to provide lots of political programming but it is only possible because of free labour and air-time. Commercial broadcasters cannot afford this kind of coverage, giving cable companies the edge. There appears to be a trend, at least in Canada, that the cable companies are looking to replace the private broadcasters as the local broadcaster as the demand for advertising revenue forces the commercial broadcasters to move from local to regional broadcasting. Since 1986 community channels have been permitted contra-advertising and sponsorship.[21] Shows with sponsorship may be chosen over those without and programmes that are likely to offend will not be aired (Layng et al 1989; CRTC 1990). Complaints have also come from the broadcast industry worried about the cable industry's unfair advantage in the competition for scarce advertising revenue.

Community access TV limits itself by following broadcast conventions. These shape the way issues are framed, and how they are treated. Broadcast TV's preoccupation with technique is unsuited to creating a public sphere for rational-critical debate. In its mimicry, community TV reinforces its secondary nature to 'real' (broadcast) television. Furthermore, the public perception of the community channel as secondary reinforces its marginal status. When there is a show of public interest, experts and leading personalities are the ones interviewed, not ordinary citizens. The community channel in Canada has become a form of 'demonstrative publicity' where public participation is seen to happen, rather than a forum of public debate wherein the public is able to represent its own interests.

> The failure of an illusion is not the failure of a
> technology ... One can read the possibilities of a medium
> only within the historical shaping that has been given to it.
> This shaping has nothing to do with an inevitable process.
>
> (Mattelart and Piemme 1980: 327)

The utopian promises have not been forgotten. In the US, many communities have had to fight for their right to a community channel, training and equipment, and many have been successful: some access channels are democratically controlled by the community, impose no censorship and have a considerable degree of public participation (Horwitz 1991). Other problems have arisen because of the limits of local government power over large cable operators, the weakness of community coalitions and problems of institutionalisation. Nevertheless, another (counter) public sphere is developing in America through satellite TV. Alternative programmes dealing with social and political issues from radical perspectives are being beamed across the US by Deep Dish TV (a coalition of arts and community groups, educational institutions and labour organisations). It broadcasts to an estimated thirty million households: probably the largest, potentially progressive, democratic public sphere ever in America's history (Deep Dish TV 1991; Dowmunt 1993).

Community television must involve the public in the management and production of programming and address itself 'to individuals as active citizens, not as consumers' (Trudel 1991: 72–3). The primary objective of cable operators is economic while the primary objective of the community channel is social; as long as these goals coincide, it is possible that a corporation may serve a community as well as a co-operatively run community channel.[22] However, if these goals conflict, the economic objectives will take precedence over the social. Nevertheless, even if the community channel is not being manipulated, the fact remains that it is open to such abuse. These problems can only be resolved by a political will to democratic control of the community channel and self-representation in the public sphere.

One final note about the introduction of 'cable access' technology was the experimentation with 'direct response' TV. This experiment began in 1974 in the US and was called Qube. What is most revealing about the Qube experiment is that it remains the primary manifestation of the real aims of the 'vested interests' behind cable TV. Qube was an experiment in home-shopping, and remains the primary motivation behind ensuring 'access' for the local communities. This example can easily be directly related to the debates about how to make the Internet pay: in the pages of the broadsheets until 1997, one could often read articles exploring the difficulties of turning the Internet into money. What has become clear is that the Internet, like community access TV, is following a similar route to radio and broadcast TV in turning into a 'licence to print money'. When that happens, the public sphere loses its 'political-ness', and its 'topicality'; it no longer functions as a proper public sphere. Community television has followed suit: most programmes are rather pleasant 'exposés' of local events, personalities and services, rather than any kind of engagement with important, relevant or topical issues.

Therefore it is possible to see that the rise of the community access TV movement began at a cross-roads between rising expectations, increased distrust of authority and the social movements which sought to engage with the authorities and the public to bring about political, economic and social change with the availability of new media technologies: cable and portapak video cameras. Nevertheless, the experience of the community and media activists in seeking access to a technological infrastructure based upon private, commercial interests regulated by the state, illustrates the hazards of the mediation of representation. While groups like Metro Media demonstrate that the possibility exists for professional and technical expertise to be harnessed for social and political organisations, the rise of a professional body of community media advisors, paid by the cable operators, demonstrates the risks of ensuring that total control remains with the industry rather than with the viewers and fee-payers. Equally important are the alternative career structures provided for people who might otherwise not have the opportunity to gain entry into the broadcasting industry, or who might use it as a stepping stone to other careers. However, such structures work against community free speech and access, especially during times of high unemployment and limited government intervention: it is much easier to ensure that representations of marginal voices and groups can be 'safe'. Yet that is not meant to be community TV's remit: its role should be to enable people to address one another about issues of public interest, and in particular it should see to it that those who are normally excluded from the mainstream public sphere should have some representation, and that representation should be in the hands of those who wish to speak.

The fact that there still remain some channels that do provide some challenging programming, aesthetically and politically, should not be overlooked, but they stand out all the more as exceptions. It should also be recognised that it is not necessarily a carefully crafted conspiracy, as a conservative impulse of not wanting to upset potential advertisers or powerful members of the community. Part of the problem with Canadian community access TV has been the institutionalising of access from the top down, which has both discouraged the activists and ensured that the cable industry maintained control over its outlets. Though no two technologies may be identical, it is clear that the democratising potential of the Internet may not be realised as long as the present unequal structures continue to privilege access for the wealthy and powerful: any technology is only as liberating as the will of the people and the social and political structures permit.

NOTES

1 Community access TV, community TV, and the community channel are used interchangeably.
2 The cable industry began in the 1950s and was initiated by a number of different individuals who wished to receive and redistribute better signals from television stations in North America.
3 This does not mean that we do not need professional media or professional communicators: but what is clear is that for far too long ordinary people have not been given many opportunities to participate, for reasons which are obvious.
4 The idea that newspaper readers do not always agree with what they read or see is sometimes used as a defence of the present set-up of newspapers.
5 The cafés, street corners and alternative media of the working class and oppositional groupings make up the counter-public sphere.
6 This is not to say that the concept does not have any problems or questions which can be raised against it, as with any methodology or theoretical framework; the advantage of the public sphere, however, is that it is a concept which is constructed out of historical study of the actual development of print and broadcast media in western European democracies (Britain, France, Germany) over the last three hundred years or so, drawing upon the insights of philosophy, the history of ideas, sociology and political science. For further critical discussions of Jürgen Habermas's concept of the public sphere, see Curran (1991), Livingstone and Lunt (1994) and especially the collection in Calhoun (1992).
7 'Active audience'studies not only show that audiences resist the dominant meanings of mass media and popular culture texts, but also that

their analyses implicitly reinforce Habermas's basic notion of the decline of the public sphere because even as audiences actively make their own meanings or resist the dominant ones there are no indications of how or where such audiences are able to connect with the public sphere (outside, perhaps, of the sub-cultural communities or identities to which they belong, which may or may not be connected to counter-public spheres). In this sense, then, these active audiences are nevertheless a 'silent' minority/majority whose resistance is not known to have any impact or intervention in the public sphere (though perhaps dominant discourses about the exclusion of women, ethnic minorities, gays and lesbians, may go some way to addressing this issue). However, these studies do not offer a way to re-think how audiences might re-connect with the public sphere.

8 It should be recognised that community access TV fell far short of its objectives but that there still survive some examples of what it could be, even if most of community TV's output is limited by the corporate, professional and governmental structures (Goldberg 1990; Surman 1997; Tuer 1994).

9 The US situation was and is very different from that in Canada (Gillespie 1975; Dolan 1984; Horwitz 1991).

10 One of the earliest American exponents was George Stoney, who had been inspired by his experience working on the CFC projects, and went on to help found the Alternate Media Center at New York University.

11 Since re-named Thunder Bay.

12 Indeed, it would appear that the CRTC is more ready to intervene against small, alternative media, such as CFRO (Co-op Radio) in Vancouver, Canada (Cook and Ruggles 1992; CRTC 1988).

13 As in the case of a radio station operator who felt it his duty to censor any news that reflected badly upon businesses advertising with the station (Hardin 1985: 23–4).

14 The four dissenting commissioners pointed out that companies like Rogers were already large enough to make the necessary capital investment in technology.

15 That is, like water, electricity, telephone or sewage, it does not make any sense to run different cables to and from every city block in order to ensure some sort of simulation of competition.

16 The acronym is based on its French name: Regroupment des Organismes Communautaires de Communication du Québec.

17 He covers the applications by community coalitions for licensing in Victoria, British Columbia and in the province of Saskatchewan. There are around six co-operative cable operators in all of Canada.

18 For example, Canadian companies have been involved in both the UK and the US.

19 It should be noted that in this programming, even if it is largely overseen and/or produced by paid staff, and few programmes are produced solely by volunteers, voluntary labour still provides the bulk of the man-hours put in to produce this programming. For example, according to an earlier study, Rogers Cablesystems' Vancouver community channel has three local neighbourhood TV outlets which

have some two or three production staff per outlet and anything from fifty to sixty volunteers each (and there is no shortage of volunteers, with a year long wait to become a volunteer being common) (Pimlott 1992).

20 Though, if there is no room for experimentation, one will never be able to find out if particular styles and genres outside mainstream broadcast standards can appeal to large audiences; indeed, where would all those 'realist', street-level dramas be today without the adoption of the supposedly amateurish, hand-held camerawork, such as that used in *NYPD Blue?*

21 Contra-advertising is a programme's acknowledgement of companies providing material support (for example, a restaurant or other location to film in, or props); sponsorship is advertising of local companies who provide funds.

22 For a comparison between the two in terms of local provision, programming and access, see Pimlott (1992).

Part II

EXCLUSION, INCLUSION AND SEGREGATION

New technology and skill in education

6

A TALE OF TWO CULTURES?

Gender and inequality in computer education

Flis Henwood, Sarah Plumeridge and Linda Stepulevage

In this chapter, the relationship between technology and inequality is critically examined through a comparison of women's experiences studying computing and information technology (IT) in two very different contexts or 'cultures' in UK higher education. The two courses examined – a traditional computer science (CS) course and an interdisciplinary (ID) IT course – are, we shall argue, representative of two opposing approaches to the problem of gender inequality in technological education. The first adopts a liberal approach and the second adopts an approach that has more in common with social constructionism. Our aims in this chapter are, first, to look at these different constructions of the 'problem' of gender inequality in relation to technology; second, to examine women's experiences in each of these computing cultures particularly in relation to their acquisition of technical skills; and, finally, to argue that a social constructionist approach would seem to be a minimum requirement for ensuring more enduring changes in gender-technology relations which leave open the possibility both of a wider range of gender positions and identities and a more progressive set of technological priorities.

Research to date has (almost universally) found that women are more attracted to computer courses that emphasise social issues and computer applications than to traditional science-based computer courses (Siann 1997). In terms of numbers alone, our research would seem to support this contention. Women constituted just 20 per cent of all CS students but over 50 per cent of ID students. In addition, women appeared to fare well, in terms of formal outcomes on both courses, but especially well on the ID course. However, in this chapter, we want to argue that, in attempting to assess the extent to which dominant gender constructions can be resisted or overturned, attention must be paid not only to formal outcomes such as pass rates, results and grades, but also more informal outcomes, including perceived levels of competence and confidence amongst the student groups. It is in assessing these levels of competence and confidence that it becomes clear how these relate to the extent to which students are able not only to acquire technical skills but to own that acquisition at a more subjective level, as part of their overall identities. We shall argue that it is this process – the 'internalisation' or 'ownership' of technical skills – that is inhibited by their continual exposure to constructions of gender-technology relations that offer women only marginal or 'outsider' status within technological cultures.

GENDER, TECHNOLOGY AND INEQUALITY

Given the falling numbers of women entering computer science at tertiary level over the last twenty years, it is not surprising that much of the research on gender and computing education to date has been driven by the desire to increase access for women to computer education, whether in schools, further, or higher education (Dain 1992; Sears 1992). However, much of this 'access' literature has tended to work with very limited and, therefore, limiting understandings of technology, of gender and of equality which rely, for the most part, on liberal discourses which incorporate a determinist model of technology and a deficit model of women and girls. In these accounts, technology (here, computers/ computing) is understood, rather unproblematically, as neutral, as simply a set of skills to be acquired. Commentators may advocate 'compensatory strategies' such as making it easier for women to 'choose' this area of study by promoting a more feminine image of computing but they tend not to question the technology as such which is perceived, in purely technical and neutral terms, as a 'given'.

Furthermore, in these accounts, women and girls are often perceived as being somehow in deficit, as needing to 'catch up' with men and boys by gaining access to this set of technical skills. Gender differences in relation to technology tend not to be addressed head-on but the implicit understanding of such gender differences is that they are largely 'added-on' and can be overcome by offering women the same opportunities as men. Here, then, gender is just a 'social distortion' underneath which there is a more neutral attribute – 'humanity', shared by men and women alike.

Thus, in liberal discourse, masculine computing and computer images are understood as cultural misrepresentation, and gender as social or cultural distortion. Underneath such distortions exist neutral technologies and equitable human relations, free of gender. Educational curricula, too, are often understood in such neutral terms. For example, the term 'hidden curriculum' is commonly used to label what are considered discriminatory practices within an otherwise neutral educational philosophy (for critique, see Bernstein 1990; Arnot 1995). Thus, it is often assumed that to bring about gender equality in education, we simply need to identify and eradicate such discriminatory practices and offer instead a gender neutral curriculum. However, as this chapter aims to show, change will not be that easy as gender-technology relations are constituted in dominant discourses and practices that are difficult to resist and challenge precisely because they impact on the construction of individuals' gender identities. Change in favour of more equitable gender relations is more likely to come about through the exploration and deconstruction of such discourses as part of the curriculum rather than through a search for a gender neutral curriculum.

As many commentators have pointed out, there are serious problems with liberal discourse and its associated 'equal opportunities' practices in the gender and technology field (Henwood 1993 and 1996; van Zoonen 1992; Grint and Gill 1995). In relation to education in particular, any such changes to the computing curriculum will necessarily be limited in that changes must not be seen to be offering anything special to women as women because emphasis on women's difference from men is seen to undermine calls for equality, which is understood, in very limited terms, as sameness (Henwood 1998). Similarly, such changes must be aimed only at finding ways of attracting women to technology as it is currently constituted and must not seek to explore, understand or challenge that constitution. Thus, apparently straightforward access and skills acquisition become the focus for liberal intervention in this field.

In addition to having a narrow understanding of the 'problem' of women and technology and hence a narrow set of 'solutions' to that problem, such approaches take little account of the potential for resistance to such interventions. Resistance may take many forms but existing research on women and technical skills suggests that such resistance may be related to the perceived threat to masculinity and dilution of status when women enter a technical field (Cockburn 1983; Hacker 1989, 1990). Indeed, this threat may explain the constant reassertion of gender difference in discourse, a process that often inhibits women's ability to speak of the contradictions they face in technological subject areas and, at the same time, hides from view the social and cultural context in which gender is actually being produced (Henwood 1998). Furthermore, it should not be forgotten that resistance may also come from women themselves who resist such compensatory strategies precisely because the changes to the curriculum that are made to 'bring women in' so often reinforce women's 'non-technical' identity.

In contrast to this liberal approach are social constructionist accounts of gender and technology relations which are less concerned with 'getting women in' to technology than with understanding why and how women are so often excluded and why technology has come to be perceived as 'masculine'. But how exactly do these social constructionist accounts deal with the question of technical skills and their acquisition, the specific focus of this chapter? First, it should be noted that, in contrast to liberal discourse, in the social constructionist literature, 'skill' is not a neutral term. Following early work by Phillips and Taylor, who argued that '[s]kill definitions are saturated with sexual bias' (1986: 55), many feminist commentators have sought to explore the ways in which, historically, male workers have managed to have their work defined as skilled, even when the content resembles women's work which is invariably defined as unskilled or semi-skilled (Cockburn 1983; Game and Pringle 1984). In this way a hierarchical gender structure is reproduced in the workplace, with men's work carrying more status than women's. Furthermore, Cockburn has shown how technology and technical skills are implicated in the very construction of gender identities so that it has become widely accepted, though not empirically proven, that men are good with technology whereas women are technically incompetent (Cockburn 1985; McNeil 1987). Gender is thus constructed, in relation to technology and technical skills, in oppositional terms, so that the acquisition of technical skills by women is perceived by many as a threat to the masculinity of men and to gender order more generally. Stepulevage (1997) builds on this analysis, arguing that women who become experts in computing are under threat of being labelled as 'other', i.e. as 'masculine' or 'lesbian', a proposition borne out by our research (see below). In the research on which this chapter is based, we were interested in examining if, and how, women experienced this binary construction on the two computer courses and what implications such constructions might have for the development of their technical skills and competences.

COMPUTER SCIENCE AND INTERDISCIPLINARY IT: TWO 'CULTURES' OF COMPUTING?

The two courses examined were taught in two different new universities in London in the early 1990s. We wanted to compare women on a conventional computer science course with those on an interdisciplinary programme, in terms of their experiences of the process of technical skills acquisition and the relative success of that process in these two very different contexts or 'cultures'. The conventional course was chosen as representative of the type of computing course few women currently choose and which is often experienced as problematic by those who do. The course was part of a programme of degrees taught within a Faculty of Science and Engineering, in the School of Computing and Information Systems. Students on all these degrees followed a largely common 'foundation' programme in their first year. From this foundation programme, we chose to focus on a module that sought to introduce students to the principles of data structures used in programming. The interdisciplinary course was chosen as indicative of a course that deliberately set out to attract women students by combining technical skills acquisition with an exploration of the social, including gender, relations of technology. This degree was taught within a Faculty of Social Sciences and comprised core and optional modules, which between them offered IT skills and contextualising studies that sought to locate and understand technologies historically, culturally and economically and with particular reference to the students' chosen specialism: education, media and communications; social research; or women and technology. Again, the students followed a common 'foundation' year and from this we chose a module offering an introduction to computers and applications software as the focus for our study.

The participants thus comprised two groups of students, studying computing in two very different contexts or cultures. We chose to focus on small groups rather than on the whole cohort for each course because we were interested in using observational and in-depth interviewing techniques (in the ethnographic research tradition) to try to understand these two cultures and these women's experiences 'from the inside', a methodology that is unworkable with large numbers of participants. The Computer Science group had sixteen students in all, of whom five were women; the Interdisciplinary group had twelve students in all, of whom five were women.[1] A combination of questionnaire and interview was used three times throughout the period of study to gather background data on the students, their reflections on the process of acquiring technical skills and on the outcomes of their study. Other data were collected via observation in workshops and seminars, examination of course documentation (validation documents, course handbooks, module handbooks and worksheets, assignment guidelines, etc.) and interviews with relevant members of staff including, where possible, those responsible for admissions, course management, module development and teaching.

How far, then, is the binary opposition of masculine/technical, feminine/non-technical in evidence in our two courses? In what ways is this opposition reproduced in discourse and practice and with what implications for female students' understanding of their own progress and outcomes? How is equality defined on each course and how does this definition fit with different understandings of gender difference? We were interested in the question of whether, where women are able to acquire technical skills and, in a formal sense, have positive outcomes, as measured by pass rates, marks, etc., it would be more difficult in some contexts than in others for them and others to recognise their skills and for them to display confidence in line with such skills acquisition. Would there, for example, be a tension between dominant discourses of gender and technology which reproduce these binary oppositions and the women's own experiences, which might suggest a greater diversity of experience? We expected such tensions would be more obvious on the traditional computer science course, closely associated with conventional masculinity, than on the interdisciplinary course where alternative discourses are promoted as part of course philo-sophy. At the very least, we expected that greater opportunities for resolution of conflict would exist on the interdisciplinary course. It is to these questions that we turn in the next section.

Computing and gender: dominant discourses

There are significant differences in the ways in which computing and technology are understood on the two courses. On the CS course, computing is defined in fairly narrow terms, in relation to professional and industrial requirements where each of the degrees will 'respond to the needs of industry in providing education that is relevant and at an appropriate state of the art (and) graduates from the scheme will continue to find a ready acceptance in industry' (CS Validation Document).

In addition, in all the CS publicity material, considerable emphasis is placed on stressing the technical facilities of the univer-sity and the specific programming languages the students will learn (Modula 2, C, Ada and PROLOG). Acquiring state-of-the-art tech-nical skills is presented as the desired outcome for CS students who seek to become professionals in the computer industry. In this discourse, the 'social' remains, typically, separate from the 'tech-nical'. For example, one tutor described the course's approach to systems design:

> We look at the practical issues in an organisation, but as a Systems Analyst you don't get involved with the political, you can't, you have to be sensitive to them but also objec-tive and don't go beyond the scope of your brief, you can't make recommendations outside of it.
> (Course Tutor, Information Systems Engineering)

In contrast, on the ID course, computing is understood in much broader terms as a technology or set of technologies that comprise technical and social aspects. The ID Validation Document describes the course as adopting 'a new approach to undergraduate education concerning technology', one in which students are encouraged to 'contextualise' new technologies via an interdisci-plinary approach which understands such technologies as innovation processes in which 'social, political, cultural, economic and tech-nical factors are interwoven'. The user is visible within this course, where great emphasis is placed on the evaluation, as well as the construction of technologies. The degree was designed around option areas that largely reflect applications areas for IT: notably Media, Education and Social Policy to ensure that technologies were evaluated in the context of their use and with user needs and requirements always in focus.

The two courses are very dissimilar. The first is a typically science-based computer course, designed to produce state-of-the-art, academically qualified and technically skilled graduates who can take their place amongst others working in the computer industry. The second is a more social science-based computer course designed to produce technically skilled users and evaluators of new IT designs and applications, with emphasis on the generic, as opposed to the specifically technical, skills acquired.

One could argue that the emphasis on science and the abstract, on the professions and on narrowly-defined technical skills and the needs of industry gives the CS course a distinctly 'masculine' feel (Kvande and Ramussen 1989; Mahoney and van Toen 1990; Verne, 1987; van Oost 1992; Stepulevage and Plumeridge 1996). In contrast, the ID course's emphasis on the social, the user and on generic technical skills and competencies gives this course a more 'feminine' feel. Indeed, in some ways, the ID course represents exactly the type of course many feminist commentators have been arguing for but, the question remains, do women necessarily fare any better on such courses and are gender and technology relations any less unequal? We will return to this question below, but first we want to look briefly at how gender and equality issues are understood on each of the courses.

On the CS course, equality and equal opportunities are understood in narrow terms as 'non-discrimination'. As the Course Tutor explained:

> Our philosophy is to teach the tried and tested methods without any bias to any particular group ... the [programming] techniques they learn have got to be the ones that are going to be effective in employment. The overall philosophy is that which industry has found most effective.

Here, we can see how equality of opportunity is understood very simply as an opportunity to acquire the skills that industry needs. Technical skills, as we saw above, are considered neutral; it is access to them that remains the area of unequal opportunity. This access can best be extended by 'non-discriminatory practices', defined here as 'treating everyone the same'. Asked if equal opportunities policies impacted on the course itself, the Course Tutor responded:

> No, I can't say we have [made changes]. We are straight down the line, but meticulously so, in that we are the *same for everyone*. I don't think I've had a discussion of lowering the criteria for certain groups of people.

It is interesting to note here that equal opportunities for women has become equated with 'lowering the criteria', again reinforcing a conception of women as less able than men in technical fields. Furthermore, and in tension with this position, it later transpired that, in an attempt to open up access to computer science, a new pathway with 'a softer name' (Software Design) had been developed and, for this pathway, there were, indeed, changed entry requirements so that science or maths A levels were no longer required (for further discussion of the significance of this development for gender equality, see Stepulevage and Plumeridge 1998).

On the ID course, by contrast, equal opportunities are part of its *raison d'être*. As argued above, social as well as technical aspects of computing were consciously built into the course design to attract those usually marginalised from technological design and decision-making: users of computer systems, women and mature students and members of the local minority ethnic communities, in particular. At least five strategies can be identified as being adopted to ensure that equal opportunities became more than a token commitment. These are:

1. targeted publicity – specifically addressing under-represented groups – and placed in minority newspapers and magazines;
2. inclusion of gender issues in core modules;
3. a specifically designed 'Women and Technology' option that provides hands-on technical skills (including database design and systems design modules) as well as an examination of the gendered relations of technology;
4. an explicit encouragement for women to select from across the full range of options and not restrict themselves to traditional areas of female employment;

119

5. the inclusion of a critical approach to designer-user relations and the re-evaluation of users' knowledge and skills, a critical pivot around which gender relations can be explored.

Thus, we could argue that whilst the CS course adopts a typically liberal approach to equal opportunities, offering no more than 'the same for all', the ID course appears to offer both a much broader interpretation of the problem and a set of practices potentially able to 'open up' and dismantle the liberal discourse, subjecting both gender and technology to much closer scrutiny within a theoretical framework closer to social constructionism. One would expect, therefore, that women would fare much better on the ID course than on the CS course and it is to this question that we now turn.

In order to compare how the two groups of women fared in terms of formal outcomes, we examined pass rates and grades for each group. However, we followed this with an analysis of data collected via observation and interview to comment on perceived levels of technical competence in the two groups. The most interesting finding here, and that which we have made the focus of this part of the analysis, is the lack of congruence between the two sets of data, pointing to issues of confidence and 'ownership' of technical skills that we relate to gender-technology relations more generally.

Formal outcomes versus perceptions of competence

Table 6.1 shows the pass rates and average grades achieved for both groups and for men and women separately.

Table 6.1 Pass rates and average marks for computer science and interdisciplinary IT groups

Group (and number in each group)	Percentage of group passing the module	Average marks for each group (expressed as percentage)
CS group (16)	56	42
CS men (11)	55	42
CS women (5)	60	43
ID group (12)	72	52
ID men (7)	50	47
ID women (5)	100	58

On the basis of these figures alone, women appear to fare better than men on both courses, although the difference is much smaller for the CS group than it is for the ID group. In addition, it appears that women on the ID course do better than women on the CS course, both in terms of the overall proportion of women successfully passing the module and the average grades achieved. The difference for men on each course is slightly in favour of CS men on pass rates but ID men on grades.

What general points can be drawn from this data and what do they tell us about gender and technology relations, more generally? The answer is, of course, very little. The sample is very small and we have followed only one year group/cohort. However, what we can say is that when formal outcomes alone are examined, women are not necessarily or, in all cases, disadvantaged on computing courses, either conventional or interdisciplinary ones. Furthermore, the data suggest that interdisciplinary courses may have something special to offer women, enabling a 100 per cent pass rate for women in this group in our study. Further analysis of the data (combined with analysis of data from other studies of this kind) would be needed before any attempt could be made to generalise these points or to identify the precise contexts within which women achieve best results. Here, our aim is to examine why, given the satisfactory and, in some cases, often excellent formal outcomes for women on these courses (i.e. their 'success' in liberal terms), these women continue to underestimate their competence in technical skills. It is to this question that we now turn.

We attempted to measure perceived levels of technical competence precisely because, following a broadly social constructionist framework, we recognised that skills are gendered and because we wanted to understand more about this gendering process. Would women continue to be defined, and to define themselves, as less technically competent than men despite evidence to the contrary on these courses? How would the gendering process differ between the two course cultures and why? The data on perceived levels of competence analysed here come from three main sources:

1. students' perceptions of their own level of competence as reflected in their answers to the following question from an interview held towards the end of their studies: 'If you had to categorise yourself in relation to technical competence now,

    how would you describe yourself (expert/technically skilled/ beginner/other)?'
2. students' perceptions of other students' technical competence from answers to the following interview question: 'Is there a particular student or students that you consider especially competent?'
3. the observer's perceptions of competence in workshops, assessed via demonstrated ability to get on alone and/or help others.

What is clear from these findings is that the women tended to underestimate their competence. In the ID group, despite accounting for four of the top five marks, the women were not confident of their skills. Two women students defined themselves as 'very poor' and 'can manage' but gained overall module grades of 60 per cent and 55 per cent and were considered competent by the observer. Another defined herself as 'a beginner' but the observer and one of the men students in her group considered her to be one of the 'experts', working well in workshops and helping others to understand. Yet another defined herself as 'knowledge-able' but the observer, and both women and men students in the group, considered her another expert. Her final grade was the highest of the group at 70 per cent. Only the self-perceptions of Student 6 matched those of both the observer and her final grade.

In contrast, the men were more mixed in their self-assessments, with four having a perception that matched other measures of competence, just one underestimating his competence and others clearly overestimating theirs. Two of the men defined themselves as 'intermediate' and 'competent and confident' but the observer saw them both as beginners and their grades were a fail and 47 per cent.

On the CS course, we see a slightly different pattern emerging. Only nine of the sixteen students in the group agreed to be inter-viewed, with probably some element of self-selection going on here.[2] Only nine students passed the module and seven of these opted to be interviewed. It may be significant for our analysis of gender-technology relations here that two of the men who failed the module agreed to be interviewed, whereas the two women who failed declined to be interviewed. So, amongst our interviewees, we had two women who were doing very well on the module and seven men, two of whom who were not progressing well. How did these students perceive themselves regarding levels of technical competence and how did such perceptions compare with the other measures of competence discussed above?

As with the ID group, women in the CS group were less confident about their technical skills than they had reason to be, as one woman achieved the joint second highest mark in the group and was considered by the observer to be one of the 'experts' in her group, and the other woman also achieved an above average grade.

The men, on the other hand, showed more confidence in themselves as technically skilled. Four of the seven described themselves as 'average' or 'expert' and three of these did, in fact, achieve grades amongst the highest in the group but, unlike the women, only one of the men – one of the two who had failed the module – showed any signs of lacking confidence in himself and his technical competence. What is particularly interesting for our analysis here is the fact that, despite achieving very similar grades to the competent men, the competent women in this group continued to feel underconfident about their technical skills. A further interesting gender difference in this group was the fact that the observed male 'expert' of the group was recognised as such by five students whereas the observed female expert went unrecognised by the students. In summary, then, women students tended to underestimate their own technical skills, both relative to other measures of their technical competence and relative to equally competent men. This was true both for the CS and the ID groups. Second, and especially for the CS course, women's expertise was less likely to be recognised than men's by other students.

It is our contention that part of the explanation for the continuing under-recognition of women's skills on these courses can be found by examining everyday discourse and practice amongst staff and students, where the binary opposition of masculine/technical, feminine/non-technical continues to be restated despite evidence to the contrary all around them.[3] In interviews, students were asked to reflect and comment upon women's under-representation in computing. Many responded using language and concepts that reflected and, at the same time, reinforced this dominant discourse. One CS student (male) commented, 'women don't like programming, and find it boring. I don't know why ... I can't visualise a woman in front of a computer writing code.' We would argue that because of this man's preconceived notions about gender and technology, reflected in the particularly strong association between men and programming, he simply cannot 'visualise a woman in front of a computer writing code'.

Other male students suggested that girls are less interested and less bothered if they cannot 'get their hands on' the computers. Typical examples here include:

> I guess boys more [*sic*] always ask for the computer, ask for games and everything and the boy always gets the computer and the girl never gets to the computer ... *she doesn't really care whether she gets to it or not.*

> I think women don't like using their brains technically and mathematically and they like theory subjects, that's the main reason.

In contrast, one of the women students says:

> Personally I find that if I have more time to play around with those little exercises they give us to do, then I become more familiar with the computer, but as it was a lot of pen and paper exercises, we didn't get very much experience on the computer which was a bit of a drag.

Despite the obvious commitment to, and interest in, computing shown in this statement, the CS women, for the most part, can be understood as confirming the gendered constructions found in dominant discourse. First, it should be noted that it proved extremely difficult to interview the women: the two 'failing' students and one other refused to be interviewed at all and the two women who were interviewed were reluctant to identify themselves with other women, preferring to interpret their experiences and strategies in terms of individual preferences and characteristics. For example, one student clearly recognises the gendered discourses of technology when she explains why she thinks women haven't gone into computing: 'Because it's a male dominated field, full stop. Men will look at you, "You're only a woman, what do you know? What are you talking about?"' However, she nevertheless continues to assume and assert a more neutral discourse when she claims that, on her course, the men treat you 'based on the amount of knowledge you've got, how much you know.' Similarly, the other woman CS student claimed that, on her Access course, she was the only woman in the class but she simply had not realised this until the teacher pointed it out to her and yet, when asked if it would have made any difference to her to have had more women on the CS course, she states 'women's attitudes are different towards things ... a lot of guys talk about computers but don't actually know much, as I found out. I think women are more hard working, including myself.' She related this hard work to the need to 'prove yourself more', a recognition of and an attempt at challenging, we would argue, the construction of women as 'technically incompetent'.

It is not that these women do not recognise some of the gendered constructions around them but that, when they recognise them, they try to overcome them in very individualistic ways by distancing themselves from 'other women' or 'women in general', thereby leaving the gendered constructions untouched. The binary oppositions operating within dominant discourses around gender and technology can actually work to silence women on technological courses who might otherwise speak of conflict and contradiction. On the other hand, it appears that these oppositions can, at times, be used by women to facilitate their learning. Gendered as non-technical, these same women told us that they expected and asked for help from tutors outside formal class times in a way that men did not.

On the ID course, although there were as many signs of the same tensions in evidence around gender and technology relations as on the CS course, there did appear to be a clearer recognition of, and more explicit reference to, the gendered nature of technology relations. Two of the women clearly recognised men's proprietorial relationship to technology:

> Men think that technology is built for them, men ... men feel superior in the sense of: 'Women shouldn't know about computers and technology.'

> I think because computing is a hard technology it's always, if you look at hard technologies, it's always men dominated [and, because of this] women need to be assertive and able to stand up for themselves and say I can do it, and work hard at getting this right because then he says, 'What do you expect, it's only a woman. She couldn't do it.'

In general, there appeared to be more space and opportunity for women on the ID course to demonstrate technical competence and expertise in the class sessions and thereby to begin to deconstruct the gendered discourses of technology. For example, there was an emphasis on collaboration and group work in workshops. This helped facilitate a display of competence and confidence by one student who adopted the role of 'substitute teacher' in her group, a role that Walkerdine (1989) has argued can be a powerful one for women in a context in which they are generally positioned as less able than men. In addition, the emphasis on the computer user on the ID course created a space in which the women students, many of whom had work experience in offices, could begin to examine and appreciate their own skills and competences. However, these spaces had to be fought for and fiercely defended in some cases, especially where men were not doing very well and felt particularly threatened by women's growing confidence. One male student, struggling in his own acquisition of technical skills, expressed his resentment and anger towards women by re-asserting the need for gender difference in a particularly aggressive manner:

> [I]t would be unfeminine because when you look at women driving HGVs [Heavy Goods Vehicles], [you might say] 'what is the difference, if a man can do it, why can't a woman?' Because (of) the hugeness of that vehicle, driven by a woman, and that woman is meant to be, you know, what should I say? I wish I had a way to class it. A woman is meant to be soft with lipstick, and you know, quite nice, easy going, but rather you see her sitting there driving a bus, to me, not other people's views, I think it's too much. I call that masculine.

Other men took issue with the provision of women-only space in the course's Women and Technology modules, attempting to undermine the women taking the option by suggesting it was the option for 'lesbians'. These 'accusations' are interesting to consider because they draw to our attention the limits of tolerance amongst men for women acquiring technical skills and encroaching, as they see it, on 'their' territories. In the mixed environment of the introductory IT module, men and women worked together and men were happy to allow women to help and guide them, especially where the women were in the fairly typical 'teacher' role, but the existence of women-only space, where women are gaining technical skills and competences for themselves alone, is perceived as much more threatening to masculinity. Maintenance of the existing gender order, it seems, requires that gender difference be always visible. Where women work separately from men, such differences cannot be readily asserted and regulated. The labelling of the Women and Technology students as lesbians suggests that the maintenance of the binary oppositions in dominant gender-technology discourse is fundamentally related to the maintenance of dominant relations of heterosexuality as well as gender (Henwood 1998; Stepulevage 1997).

MOVING ON: RETHINKING GENDER EQUALITY IN TECHNOLOGY RELATIONS

Although the numbers involved in this study are very small, the detailed qualitative data analysis undertaken (some of which forms the basis for this chapter) does appear to suggest that there is some mechanism at work which continues to re-assert dualistic gender categories and identities in gender-technology relations, despite what would otherwise be very convincing evidence of the potential for their demise.

The relationship between gender and technical expertise has been explored in various ways in the gender and technology literature, most often with women being understood as actively excluded from technology and technical expertise but the analysis given here suggests a slightly different understanding is needed. Women in our research were not being denied access to technical skills in any formal sense. On the CS course, although the proportion of women is low, women's formal outcomes (marks and pass rates) are no worse than men's, and on the ID course they fare better than men on these measures. However, what our analysis does suggest is that, despite having reason to be as confident about technical skills and competence as the equivalent group of men, women in our research groups continue to underestimate their skills and continue to equate technical competence and skill with masculinity and men.

In dominant cultural representations, men and women are constructed in oppositional terms: men as 'good' with technology, women as technically 'incompetent', but these representations, rather than being accepted as reflective of some 'reality' or 'truth' about men's and women's attributes, instead need to be understood as part of the broader picture of gendered discourse that surrounds technology relations and that positions men and women so differently.

What this research demonstrates is that to fail to understand the social and cultural nature of the gender-technology relationship will result in aborted attempts at change in those relationships. In contexts like our CS course that operate with a very liberal under-standing of equal opportunities, both 'gender' and 'technology' are taken at face value and their cultural nature is not understood. This limits the space that exists within such courses for students (or staff) to examine the gendered relations of technology and the resistances to change in those relations. The broader understanding of gender-technology relations on the ID course opens up some spaces in which the cultural nature of those relations can be explored, deconstructed and challenged. However, this 'alternate' discourse does not exist in isolation and students (and staff) have to negotiate their way through the conflict posed by the intersec-tion of this discourse with more traditional discourses that reassert binary oppositions, continuing to equate technical competence with men and leaving women marginalised and 'outsiders' in tech-nological culture.

NOTES

1 These proportions are not representative of the course cohorts overall, where women represented 20 per cent of all the CS students and over 50 per cent of the ID students. Thus, our research groups (at about 30 per cent and 40 per cent women, respectively) over-represent women on the CS course and under-represent them on the ID course.
2 See Stepulevage (1997), for a fuller discussion of this aspect.
3 Further discussion of the workings of this discourse in the CS course can be found in Stepulevage and Plumeridge (1998).

7

TENDING TO THE TAMAGOTCHI

Rhetoric and reality in the use of new technologies for distance learning

Nod Miller, Helen Kennedy and Linda Leung

In this chapter we reflect upon our experience of Project @THENE (Accessing Technology for Higher Education and New Enterprise), a distance learning programme designed to enhance access to information technology-related higher education for mature black women, which uses the multimedia technologies which are its subjects of study as one of the modes of delivery. We consider the extent to which the use of new technologies for educational purposes may contribute to the breaking down of social inequalities in access to higher education and in relation to the acquisition of technical knowledge and skills. We contrast the rhetoric in current educational policy documents about new technologies and social change with our experience of using new technologies for educational purposes, pointing to the considerable challenges and tensions – economic, technical and pedagogic – faced by learners and tutors attempting to operate in a virtual learning community. The image of tending to the tamagotchi arose in a project meeting where a colleague likened the needs within a distance learning group to those of her son's electronic pet, for which she was responsible during school hours.

TECHNOLOGIES AND INEQUALITIES IN PROJECT @THENE

@THENE was a BT (British Telecom)-funded pilot project in which we aimed to enhance access to university courses in new technology through the establishment of a foundation course delivered partly by distance learning through multimedia technologies. The project incorporates a partnership between the University of East London and a local education and training centre (NEWTEC). In Project @THENE, the fourteen students who participated in the pilot year accessed teaching materials and communicated with tutors responsible for the distance learning element of the course through computers which were installed in their homes. The project also involved researching the ways in which communication is conducted in a distance learning environment and attempting to assess the strengths and weaknesses of various media for course delivery.

A further aim of Project @THENE was to implement teaching about multimedia technologies by using the technologies which formed the content of the curriculum as modes of delivery. This dual role for computer technology has been the source of some of the difficulties we have encountered during Project @THENE. The curriculum of @THENE was made up of the following four units:

Unit A: Technology in Society
Unit B: The Computer, Inside and Out: how to use it and how it works
Unit C: Learning to Learn: preparing for higher education
Unit D: Exploring Technology: bringing it all together.

Unit D was taught completely at a distance and some elements of Unit C were also taught in this way. Units A and B were taught face-to-face. As Unit D took up 50 per cent more time than the other individual units, this meant that about half of @THENE students' studies were carried out at a distance and it is this aspect of the @THENE course with which we are concerned in this paper. Helen Kennedy was a researcher and the distance learning tutor on @THENE; Linda Leung was researcher, Unit B tutor and provided some technical support to the project; Nod Miller was project director.

Project @THENE and the @THENE course both developed out of a face-to-face Year Zero course which has been delivered for four years at the time of writing. This face-to-face version of Year Zero (named TOPs – Taught on the Premises – by the students themselves) continued to run during the pilot year of @THENE and thus formed a control group for our research.

The project aimed to take action in relation to a range of inequalities, as the students on @THENE were all women from ethnic minority backgrounds, all were mothers, many were single parents and all but one lived in east London, which has been described as 'one of the most remarkably underdeveloped and deprived zones in the affluent South East [of England]' (Hall 1991: 7) due to its economic disadvantage, recent de-industrialisation and high unemployment, which extends to 40 per cent of the economically active amongst ethnic minority communities in some boroughs in the region. In many senses then, the project was trying to address educational inequality. @THENE students come from groups who have been disadvantaged in respect of access to higher education as well as to knowledge about and use of information technology (IT), so the project was also addressing questions about inequality in relation to technology. In attempting to widen access to higher education for mature black women (a group particularly under-represented in the university sector), we are addressing a problem identified as a priority by policy-makers. However, our preliminary findings indicate that attempting to counter inequality in this way is no easy task.

THE HUNGER OF THE TAMAGOTCHI

The idea for this paper developed out of a discussion in a project meeting where we were reviewing recent progress of students on the @THENE programme and exchanging stories about tutors' interactions with students. One colleague enumerated the many phone calls and e-mails she had sent and received over the previous fortnight, expressing concern about how to deal appropriately with the messages received from students. We hypothesised that the hunger for support (technical, economic, pedagogical and emotional) from students was ultimately insatiable, given our finite resources. We noted that although the grant from BT enabled us to contribute to students' telephone bills as well as to provide computer equipment, students had still further needs; a colleague reported that one of the @THENE students had requested that the university provide her with office furniture in order to facilitate her use of the computer. We also noted that, however many hours of tutor time were dedicated to student support in the distance learning unit of the course, the level of provision was nevertheless sometimes insufficient to meet the students' needs. Members of the project team commented on the tendency for government policy statements on education to imply that practical problems in using technology were non-existent or easily soluble.

At this point a colleague's briefcase began to emit loud squeaking noises. The owner of the briefcase pulled out a small piece of digital technology and pressed some buttons on its miniature keyboard. She explained that the alarm noises reminded her to administer treatment to her son's tamagotchi. A tamagotchi is an electronic pet whose virtual existence needs to be maintained by human intervention; buttons must be pressed at intervals to simulate feeding, cleaning, cuddling and giving medicine if the creature is to survive. Our colleague explained that these creatures were hugely popular among schoolchildren and that they had caused such consternation and havoc in classrooms (particularly when they died) that most of the local schools had banned them from school premises. Her son had now given her charge of his electronic animal during school hours; he had been distraught when the creature starved to death while his mother was in a meeting and she was therefore anxious not to have this second pet die again whilst in her charge.

This incident led into a discussion of the metaphor of the tamagotchi during which a colleague remarked on the aptness of the image of the digital creature as constantly hungry and needy in capturing the capacity of technology to create the need for more, rather than less, human effort to be expended in some contexts. The squeaks of the tamagotchi for attention seemed to embody the cries of the adult distance learner for more resources, more equipment and more pastoral support. In our attempt to use technologies to overcome educational inequality we have found that our distance learning students, like tamagotchis, have required constant, labour-intensive care and attention.

In this chapter we identify specific incidents in our experience of Project @THENE which illustrate some of the economic, technical, pedagogic and interpersonal challenges which we faced in our attempts to counter inequalities in relation to knowledge and control of technologies of networked and multimedia computing. We set our experience against the background of current state policy in the UK in respect of the use of information and communication technologies in adult and higher education and draw out some possible implications of our experience for this policy and for pedagogic practice in distance education.

ASSUMPTIONS ABOUT TECHNOLOGY IN EDUCATIONAL POLICY DOCUMENTS

In 1997, shortly after the election of a New Labour government, a number of policy documents were published which indicated the likely direction of educational change at the beginning of the twenty-first century. Documents particularly relevant to adult and higher education, the sectors with which we are concerned in this project, include the Dearing Report on higher education (DfEE 1997a), the Fryer Report (*Learning in the Twenty-First Century* 1997), and the DfEE's consultation paper on lifelong learning (*The Learning Age: a renaissance for a new Britain* 1998). These papers stress the importance of widening participation in higher education and encouraging partnerships between universities and other providers of learning opportunities, and embody the belief that increased use of new technologies for teaching and learning can make an important contribution to these goals.

Some of the ways in which the present government expects new technologies to transform education are set out in the consultation paper on the National Grid for Learning, which sets out proposals for the development of 'a mosaic of inter-connecting networks and education services based on an Internet which will support teaching, learning, training and administration in schools, colleges, universities, libraries, the workplace and homes' (DfEE 1997b: 3).

The authors of the paper clearly believe that the establishment of the Grid will bring about improvements in the quality and efficiency of school-based education, and suggest major implications for teaching and learning, staff development and administration in the projected increase in the use of information and communication technologies (ICTs) in education.

One of the themes which runs through the Dearing Report is the potential for the innovative use of ICTs to improve the quality and flexibility of higher education and its management. The authors of the Report believe that such usage gives scope for a reduction in costs, although they do acknowledge that 'in the short term, implementation requires investment in terms of time, thought and resources' (DfEE 1997a: Section 65). They recommend that all higher education institutions in the UK should have in place over-arching communication and information strategies by 1999/2000, suggesting that the main challenges for the future are to harness the UK's existing information technology infrastructure and to ensure the production of high quality materials and good management of educational and technological systems, in order to meet the needs of students and other clients. They state that 'students will soon need their own portable computers as a means of access to information and for learning via a network' (DfEE 1997a: Section 65) and 'that students will need access to high quality networked desktop computers that permit the use of the latest multimedia materials and other applications' (DfEE 1997a: Section 65). Recommendation 46 of the report is as follows: 'We recommend that by 2000/1 higher education institutions should ensure that all students have open access to a Network Desktop Computer, and expect that by 2005/06 all students will be required to have access to their own portable computer' (DfEE 1997a: Section 68).

The authors of the Fryer Report predict that universities and colleges are likely to see the enormous growth of part-time study, distance learning and technology-based programmes. They see universities as having a particularly important part to play in developing expertise in these areas and applaud the principle of universities and other educational providers and learners working in close partnership with one another to provide flexible, technology-based systems of learning. Fryer and his colleagues are clearly excited by what they refer to as 'the digital revolution' which they see as offering the opportunity for active learning via multimedia technologies and they state that:

> New digital technologies will create learning opportunities which are not dependent on being available at a particular time or place. Learning at home and outside conventional educational establishments will become more widespread – with implications for institutions, teachers and content creators (like broadcasters) as well as individual learners. Tailoring resources to individual needs will eventually become possible.
>
> (Fryer 1997: 15.5)

They recommend that the government should adopt policies to secure access to new technologies, such as Internet connectivity or access for everyone, including those for whom financial barriers would otherwise be insuperable. In addition, they stress the importance for government, funders and providers to establish arrangements to encourage individuals to acquire relevant skills and knowledge (Fryer 1997: 15.10).

The Learning Age, which draws on the Fryer Report, gives less detailed attention than Fryer to the use of technology for learning, although the authors of this Green Paper do assert that 'one of the best ways to overcome some of the barriers to learning will be to use new broadcasting and other technologies. We expect their role in learning more generally to increase significantly.' (DfEE 1998: 22). It is suggested that the proposed University for Industry will promote good practice in the use of new technologies for teaching and learning, and that broadcasters are to be encouraged to become more centrally involved in the provision of learning materials, with the availability of new digital broadcasting channels opening up opportunities for increased educational delivery. Discussions are promised with broadcasters and cable providers to explore ways in which their programme-making facilities and digital networks could support interactive learning, although it is not made clear in *The Learning Age* (DfEE 1998) where the motivation will come from for commercial companies in the ICT industries to involve themselves in educational provision.

The writers of policy documents such as these would no doubt acknowledge that their recommendations raise more questions than are answered about how new technologies are best to be used to achieve broad educational goals. But it is not too difficult to distil some of the assumptions in these papers regarding the relationship of technology to education and the direction of developments in this field over the next decade if not the next millennium. Despite the importance assigned to technology, the term is seldom if ever defined or seen as problematic; its usage seems most often to connote hardware and there is relatively little mention of technological skills or knowledge other than occasional mentions of the need for students to acquire keyboard skills. This narrow definition of technology contrasts with the view widely expounded by sociologists of technology that technology should be seen as comprising physical objects, the knowledge required to use them and the knowledge required to create them (MacKenzie and Wajcman 1985: 3–4).

The use of new technologies generally seems to be seen as a key feature of a 'learning society' where all may be learners, where all may study where and what they want, and where a system of mass higher education offers choice, flexibility, quality and coherence. Subtextual images which hang under the measured prose of the policy documents are those of technology as either hard and heavy or invisible and magical. Another subtextual element is a belief in the determining, causal nature of technology. For example, digital technologies are seen as having the power to transform distance learning, enabling geography, space and time to be manipulated and managed in ways which benefit learners and cut costs.

The statements made in policy documents such as the ones to which we have referred in this brief sketch need to be seen as both informing and being informed by other public debates, such as those conducted in academic and scientific communities and in news and current affairs programmes and publications, about technology and education. In an earlier paper (Miller, Leung and Kennedy 1997) we discussed the polarity which we noted in the academic literature on technology and learning between utopian and dystopian discourses: between those who view the use of new technologies in education with great optimism and those who are convinced that growing use of technology will increase social divisions and inequalities. Recent government policy statements have generally been constructed within the utopian discourse. We have attempted in Project @THENE to negotiate the boundaries between extremes of technophilia and technophobia and of evangelical enthusiasm and Luddite despair. In offering a critical perspective on the assumptions and subtexts which we read in the policy documents, and in setting out elements in our experience of this particular case study, we are aware that that our analysis may be read as pessimistic. We would not want this to be seen as our definitive style or location but we see this emphasis as necessary in order to counterbalance dominant discourses of technology and education as represented in policy documents.

In the sections which follow, we contrast our experience in Project @THENE with the rhetoric of educational policy statements, identifying the tension which exists between the university's objective to introduce more flexible forms of educational delivery and the constraints upon resources which make it difficult to support such initiatives.

TECHNO-ECONOMIC ISSUES

Popular conceptualisations of virtual learning communities emphasise the learning opportunities offered to those who may otherwise not participate in higher education, but seem to ignore the high level of resourcing required. While distance learning is being championed as the solution to ensuring access to higher education, the evidence from Project @THENE suggests that this can only be done where there are considerable subsidies for the technology and technical support. Our experience in this project demonstrates that educational inequality cannot be tackled through technology alone, but requires economic and human resources to build and support a technical infrastructure.

The computer hardware and software on which part of @THENE's course delivery depended was purchased with project funds provided by BT and was subsequently loaned to students for the duration of the one-year course. The installation and rental of additional telephone lines for Internet access was also funded by the project. Online time of two to nine hours per week was subsidised, as were a limited number of telephone calls between students and to tutors at the university. Without this level of financial assistance, it is clear that few if any of the students would have been able to afford to undertake this mode of study and we took these measures out of a recognition of and an attempt to address the socio-economic disadvantage of these students.

As we have indicated, the Dearing Report suggests that employing technology and flexible modes of educational delivery will not only address unequal participation in higher education, but reduce costs as well. When the economics of employing new technologies in education have been considered, the transition from traditional face-to-face teaching methods to open and flexible computer-mediated distance learning may not be as smooth as the policy-makers envisage. There is a discrepancy between those who claim that only an initial investment is needed in the short term to achieve economies of scale in the long term, and the practice on @THENE of the necessary, ongoing and additional administration involved in ensuring that telephone bills were paid on time and that students did not exceed their subsidy as well as in liaising with the university's finance department and with the telephone company and there is no reason to believe that the need to carry out these tasks would disappear if the project were to continue running in future years. The increase in the administrative load was not accompanied by any immediately evident decrease in the time spent dealing in pedagogic activities, so that so far we have little indication of any reduction in costs.

Consequently these administrative responsibilities which have been a necessary part of the delivery of the @THENE course have raised questions about the supposed cost savings associated with distance learning. Indeed, one particular incident showed that the financial consequences of this mode of delivery are difficult to control where flexibility is an inherent part of the course and the explicit aim is to widen access to higher education.

Students were informed at the outset of the @THENE course that it was their responsibility to keep a record of their online time, to submit their bills promptly for payment, to ensure that the costs of their online time remained within the subsidy if they could not afford to pay the excess, or to pay the additional costs if the subsidy was exceeded. Three months before the completion of the course, one student submitted an expensive telephone bill which meant that she had nearly used all her subsidy. She admitted that she would not have the funds to pay any amount over and above the subsidy. Thus, she was faced with the choice of restricting her use of the Internet for the remainder of the course to the point where this might be insufficient for her to complete her coursework properly or continuing her high levels of Internet usage and finding some way of meeting the additional costs. However, there were no mechanisms in place for policing or restricting students' Internet access or for dealing with students who subsequently could not or would not pay outstanding amounts on their telephone bills. Although the university was only subsidising students' online time, it was ultimately responsible for the telephone lines as it had authorised and paid for their installation.

Such incidents have potentially serious financial implications and are therefore a constant cause of concern. This specific incident exemplifies our two central findings in relation to the economics of computer-mediated distance education: that it is expensive and that its costs are difficult to predict and control. Our experience therefore leads us to question Fryer's contention that through the use of ICTs access to higher education can be widened to facilitate 'enormous growth' while addressing learning requirements individually or 'tailoring resources to individual needs', particularly if it is assumed that at least some students will be on very low incomes. Many of the costs of providing learning through networked computers are not immediately obvious, particularly to middle-class people who do not generally lose sleep over the size of their telephone bills. The costs of line installation and rental are likely to be prohibitive for many students and there are other hidden costs such as the annual fees to be paid to providers of technical support as well as insurance and replacement costs of software and hardware.

The economics of Project @THENE are often enmeshed in other aspects of delivery, particularly technical issues. As a pilot study, the findings of the project may be used to adapt this mode of educational delivery on a wider scale to other courses across the university. However, even with the small number of students participating in the project, the capacity to provide technical support extended beyond the scope of the course delivery team, the department administering the course and indeed, the university's information technology (IT) department. The IT department's responsibilities include technical support to staff, but not students; and maintenance of the university's computer equipment on campus, but not that which is off-site. Clearly, the success of @THENE's computer-mediated distant delivery would depend on a well-supported technical infrastructure. Therefore, technical support for Project @THENE was provided externally by an organisation which is typically contracted to assist commercial environments. Its clients are usually companies in which staff are centrally located and skilled in the use of computers. By contrast, no computer experience whatsoever was assumed of @THENE students, who were studying in their homes in disparate locations at times which might be out of office hours. The educational market was a new departure for the organisation, making it difficult to cost the service they would eventually provide for the project. Nonetheless, it regarded Project @THENE as providing a good opportunity to gain experience in providing technical support to the education sector, given that this might be potentially lucrative for the company in the future with the increasing adoption of distance learning methods. The need to venture outside the university for support of this kind highlights the inequalities in technical resources, knowledge and power which exist between the education sector and the private sector. The university, with its limited resources, could not provide the level of support necessary; although a commercial organisation could, its primary interest is in generating profit. This profit-making imperative means that projects which aim to widen access to higher education which purchase the services of these companies are unlikely to result in a reduction in the costs of educational provision.

The service that the organisation provided was essentially the same as that given to its commercial clients. Technical support was available during normal business hours only, with problems initially logged by telephone. Where possible, technical problems were resolved by remote access. Otherwise, an engineer was dispatched to the student's home. The organisation was paid an agreed lump sum for the provision of this service. However, at a review meeting six months into the project, the organisation declared that it was no longer commercially viable to give technical assistance to @THENE students as their relative inexperience in the use of IT meant that many and frequent requests for support had been made, far more than had been anticipated. Consequently, the organisation wanted additional remuneration to continue the service. Without the service, students' progress on the course would have been severely inhibited if a technical problem should arise. Yet the project did not have sufficient funds to ensure the continued provision of this level of support. In the event, the company did continue to provide support and, predictably, rather less support was needed in the latter phases of the project as students' skills and confidence with their computers increased.

This illustrates the dilemmas of attempting to address unequal access to higher education through technology-mediated distance learning in the context of limited funds and constraints on resources. It demonstrates that an adequately supported technical infrastructure is needed, but contrary to much of the rhetoric about distance learning and technology in education, this does not come cheaply, particularly where it is provided by a commercial enterprise. However, the constraints on resources within educational institutions make it difficult to provide such support in-house even though it may be more cost-effective. But educational policy still seems to be focused on technology in itself, failing to consider that more than just 'access to high quality networked desktop computers' (DfEE 1997a: Sections 65–8) is required to encourage participation in higher education which is representative of the wider community.

The @THENE experience also offers a cautionary note in relation to the claims that technology in education effectively empowers students. One of our aims in Project @THENE was to increase women's participation in the use of new technologies, in order to contribute to counteracting the gender inequalities in IT occupations and training. Project @THENE attempted to push back the boundary delineating who may acquire knowledge of new technologies, and to create conditions under which this knowledge was made more readily accessible to women than has tended to be the case in the past: the general absence of women from the institutions which define and create technology and the exclusion of women from fields such as computing and microelectronics have been well documented (see, for example, Cole et al 1994; DP Connect 1997; Karpf 1987; Linn 1987; Spender 1996). However, we have found that the provision of external technical support is almost entirely male-dominated. The opportunities for @THENE's mature women students to learn through use about technology arise in the face of the male technical support engineers who are the gatekeepers to the technology and have the power to define who is 'at fault'. On a number of occasions, the organisation resisted providing technical support on the basis of an assumption that the student, being a woman, was not competent with the equipment and therefore likely to be responsible for the given technical problem. When 'user fault' was deemed to be the case, the organisation argued that it should charge a fee for each on-site visit to students' homes. The combination of technical, economic, social and gender considerations constantly pervaded the delivery of the @THENE Year Zero, indicating that the role of new technologies in resolving educational inequalities may be much more complex than policy-makers ever imagined.

PEDAGOGIC ISSUES

Practical experience on Project @THENE has raised our awareness of some pedagogical issues in computer-mediated distance learning. The project started with the design of the @THENE course, the distance learning element of which was influenced by two key issues in distance education. One assumption about distance education that we came across in the preparatory phase of Project @THENE is that it involves learning that students undertake 'on their own'. At the internal validation meeting of @THENE, one senior member of university staff sought to clarify his understanding of the course's structure by asking if Unit D was the unit where 'students are left on their own' and other colleagues expressed similar concerns about the isolation that they understood distance learning students experience. We approached the design of Unit D with the belief that feelings of isolation were not inevitable features of distance learning and we tried to devise strategies to overcome these feelings. We incorporated tasks which involved regular, different types of communication, both synchronous and asynchronous, into the course materials. In the early stages of the course, this included, for example, telephone conferences; paired and small group work to be completed face-to-face, on the telephone or via e-mail; summaries of completed tasks to be e-mailed to all students; communication structures in which A sends a message to B, B sends a message to C and so on; and online interviews conducted by students with each other. In the later stages, students' tasks included experimenting with newsgroups, online conferences, MUDs and other forms of networked communication. Although they communicated primarily amongst themselves, they also made contact with a range of other people online.

In order for the communication to be effective, students needed to do the work at roughly, although not exactly, the same time. For this reason, the unit was divided into blocks, each block was broken down week-by-week (this was not unique to Unit D: all other units were broken down in the same way) and students were encouraged to try to manage their time so that they completed each weekly activity on time. Activities were distinct from assessed assignments; they replaced the classroom-based discussions that take place during a face-to-face course of study. For example, in a block about the Internet, students were asked to review what they had learnt by designing five interview questions and carrying out e-mail interviews with each other in pairs. In a later block about uses of networks, three @THENE newsgroups were set up: a classroom, where structured activities took place; a newsroom, which was used to exchange information, tips and news; and a coffeeroom, which tutors did not enter and which students were subsequently free to use as they chose. In addition, Helen, the tutor for the distance learning unit, tried to ensure that she sent e-mail messages to the whole group and to individuals each week; throughout most of the course, she telephoned students if she had not heard from them by e-mail for a couple of weeks. These are just some examples of the different types of communication that were built in to Unit D to try to minimise experiences of isolation amongst students.

One of the key strengths of distance learning is the flexibility that it brings with it: this is often one of the reasons why this delivery method is adopted. In distance learning, tutor and student do not need to be in the same place at the same time in order for education and communication to take place. At the outset of our project we believed that this flexibility would help @THENE widen access to education for mature women: women with domestic responsibilities or a need to take employment outside the home could fit their studies around their other duties. In practice this assumption was confirmed, as a number of @THENE students felt they would be unable to study on a fully face-to-face basis. The structure of @THENE has meant that students were able to carry out their studies late at night when their children were in bed: Helen has received e-mail sent at all hours of the morning and night, for example at 4:27am, when most of us are asleep, and at 6:58am, before most of us have woken up. Other students were employed outside the home on the days that they did not attend college and they too completed their studies late at night or at the weekend.

However, the decision to structure Unit D on a week-by-week basis and incorporate regular communication meant that the degree of flexibility in the unit was limited: students could work at any time of the day or night, but they were expected to complete a task by a given deadline. We saw this as a compromise, which made it possible to find a way both to minimise isolation and to make use of the flexibility distance learning provides. However, within the formal structures of a degree programme, flexibility is somewhat restricted. For example, within @THENE we took the decision that students would still need to complete assessment by given dates in order to progress to the next level, and in this sense a degree of inflexibility existed within the programme.

In the interview and selection process for the @THENE course, we asked candidates what they thought the advantages and disadvantages of distance learning might be, in order to help us select those candidates who were best suited to and prepared for the @THENE model of delivery. When the course started, in order to prepare chosen candidates, now @THENE students, for their distance learning experience, the first two weeks of Unit D were taught on a face-to-face basis. In these sessions we discussed what it meant to be a distance learning student and to have a computer in the home and how students would need to organise their work, their homes and their lives in order to succeed on @THENE. The distance learning tutor felt that these discussions were productive, as students considered some of the problems that might arise whilst studying at home, identified where to go for help, shared ideas and identified each other as important sources of support.

Throughout the duration of @THENE, few students consistently completed tasks by the given deadlines. On average, about half of the students completed tasks more or less within the time frame, give or take a few days, with only one student consistently completing the work before the specified deadline. It was not uncommon for students to fail to do the work at all, particularly when tasks did not form the basis of formal assessment. For example, four out of fourteen students submitted complete notes from their paired interviews in which they reviewed their learning in the block about the Internet and two more students completed part of this activity. Another example is of synchronous newsgroup discussions for which students had been arranged into three groups of four in advance (one student was ill at the time and another was abroad). Of the first group, three out of four participated, with one of these three joining late; of the second group, two out of four participated; of the third, one participated throughout, one joined late and another tried to join late, but sent her messages as e-mail, not newsgroup messages, which were consequently not received in the newsgroups. These latter two attempted to join late after Helen had rung them up to remind them of the activity. Consequently, of fourteen students, five participated fully, two partially and one attempted but failed to participate in this activity.

Despite our best efforts to design Unit D in such a way that facilitated students' successful completion, we found that distance learning was experienced as challenging and painful for @THENE students. Discussions with students about why they sometimes failed to complete distance learning activities revealed a range of reasons: housing problems, students' own and their dependants' illness, financial problems, technical problems, lack of practice in time-management and failure to acknowledge distance learning tasks as equally important as other activities have all been cited by students as explanations. Some of these are beyond the scope of the course, although we talked to students about how they might impact on their studies; others seem related to the difference between distance learning and other types of learning and suggest that while some students managed to become successful independent learners, others did not. Whether anything else could have been done at interview or in induction to prepare @THENE students better to cope with the distance learning element of their studies is a question which deserves further reflection.

The pedagogic issues raised by Project @THENE underline the central argument of this paper: there is no simple technical fix to the problems of educational inequality. Educational challenges do not disappear when teaching and learning move out of the class-room and into a virtual environment: rather, the problems faced by learners and tutors in face-to-face settings may be amplified in the course of electronic communication and course delivery. Our experience of @THENE has led us to confront some difficult questions about how we manage interpersonal communication inside a virtual classroom or learning community; we have become increasingly aware of the care required in managing electronic communication, and of the need to recognise the possibility of differences of assumption, affective reaction and meaning arising in the course of e-mail interaction. We expect these issues to continue to preoccupy us in relation to our practice as educators well into the future.

CONCLUSIONS

Like the tamagotchi, many of the @THENE distance learning students needed a lot of tending. The nature of the Year Zero course is such that it will attract students with a range of personal circumstances which present obstacles to successful study, whether these be financial constraints, health problems, or lack of practice in the art of studying. This means that in order to overcome educational inequalities for the social groups with which we are concerned, significant resources are needed. It may be that this will not be the case with all student groups. In Project @THENE we have learned that the use of new technologies in course delivery does not offer any magic: technological solutions can be costly and imperfect as technologies sometimes fail to work, and it is not surprising to learn that the problems that exist in classroom-based courses do not disappear in the virtual learning community. The prospect of intervention through educational practice in relation to geography, space, time is quite breathtaking, but since we were also attempting in this project to wrestle with poverty, racism and sexism as well, it may well be that we were attempting too much innovation at once.

We challenge the optimism of the rhetoric about new technologies, as our experience has revealed a number of practical difficulties, personal uncertainties and ideological tensions in using

new technologies to overcome inequalities which the policy statements generally fail to recognise. We feel it is important to expose
some of the myths that surround the potential of new technologies
and therefore we have tended to concentrate on the difficulties we
have encountered on Project @THENE. In doing this, we do not
wish to give the impression that @THENE has been without its
successes: all but three @THENE students progressed into Year
One of the degree programme and have expressed their own sense
of success in terms of what they have learnt about new technologies during @THENE. Similarly, as a research project, @THENE
has been tremendously productive, generating a vast range of
learning and research data.

Part III

TECHNOLOGY, INEQUALITY AND ECONOMIC DEVELOPMENT

8

SOCIAL INEQUALITY, TECHNOLOGY AND ECONOMIC GROWTH

Chris Freeman

This chapter is in four parts. The first part introduces the idea of long swings in policies dealing with social inequality over half a century or more. It describes, in particular, the role of one ardent social reformer in Britain – Eleanor Rathbone – because of her exceptional importance in the evolution of what became the 'Welfare State'. Reformist policies for social services and redistribution of income seem to alternate with periods of reversal and retrenchment. The second part of the chapter suggests that these long swings in social policy and in income distribution have some connection with long cycles in the economy – the so-called 'Kondratieff waves'. The third part tries to show how and why the trend towards greater inequality emerges when a major new technology is spreading through the economic system. The fourth part shows how this inequality also manifests itself in the wealth and poverty of whole nations, through the uneven development of the world economy. Finally, the conclusions suggest very briefly some ways in which the present trends towards greater inequality with all their dangerous social and political consequences might be reversed.

LONG SWINGS IN SOCIAL POLICY AND INEQUALITY

Concern with social inequality is a recurrent theme of British political life and indeed of world politics. Ever since the Old Testament prophets, if not earlier, many people have found something

149

morally repulsive about the co-existence of extremes of wealth and poverty, especially when the highest incomes and the largest fortunes were not earned by hard work or by exceptional creativity. This ethical concern has been periodically reinforced by fear and by prudence – the fear of rebellions and social unrest and prudence in attempting to avert rebellion by timely reforms. Although seldom if ever approaching a truly egalitarian distribution of income and wealth, which was in fact rarely advocated by anyone, except by George Bernard Shaw in the 1890s and some of the Levellers in the 1640s, these pressures did lead periodically to a wave of social reforms which mitigated the worst hardships in the lives of the poor and the socially excluded (to use today's fashionable terminology). Even if these reforms were sometimes not sufficient to reverse a general trend towards greater inequality, they did provide some temporary alleviation.

In the 1980s and 1990s it has sometimes seemed that both the ethical concern and even the prudence had disappeared. In Britain and the United States especially, but also in many other European countries, the trend of fiscal policy which had been flowing strongly in favour of progressive taxation since the Second World War was reversed. After the war, high levels of taxation on high incomes had been widely advocated and accepted as the norm. Moreover, the gap between skilled and unskilled wages was drastically reduced during and after the war. So general was this trend that Williamson and Lindert, historians of wealth and poverty in the United States, committed themselves in 1980 to this generalisation: 'In contrast with the previous periods of wealth levelling, the twentieth century levelling has not been reversed' (Williamson and Lindert 1980: 33).

Unfortunately for their generalisation, very soon afterwards, of course, it was reversed, not only in the United States but worldwide. Even in countries like Sweden, fiscal regimes were modified in a regressive direction and the biggest changes of all came in the former Communist countries, from a rather egalitarian distribution of income to an extremely unequal distribution (and often no income at all for the poorest). This trend has also been strong in countries like China, which have remained nominally Communist, whilst moving towards free market economies. In the UK, the share of the lowest 20 per cent of household disposable incomes fell from 10 per cent in 1979 to 6 per cent in 1992, while the share of the top 20 per cent rose from 35 to 43 per cent (CSO 1995: Table 5.19). That was a pretty drastic and rapid change in the

150

space of little more than a decade in the 1980s, brought about mainly by a combination of mass unemployment on the one hand and big tax reductions for the rich on the other. In the 1990s, the reduction in unemployment in the United States and the UK brought about some improvement in the situation but no major redistributive tax changes were brought into effect.

Indeed, the British government set its face firmly against a return to redistributive taxation and embraced the objective of 'reforming' the welfare state. It is not yet clear in what direction all these reforms might go – which benefits might be reduced and which might be increased and which eliminated entirely. However, the episode of the single mothers did not augur well for those who supposed that a Labour government might move in the direction of the Liberal Government of 1906 or the Labour Government of 1945, both of which introduced reforms which later came to be known collectively as the 'Welfare State'. However, the 1998 and 1999 Budgets did include some measures with mildly redistributive effects, so it is worth recalling some of the main principles of the Welfare State and how they were viewed by its leading advocates in relation to inequality. Questions of gender, of employment and of health were all considered to be fundamental and inter-connected by Sir William Beveridge when his committee drafted their Report in 1941–2. The emphasis on family allowances must be attributed primarily to Eleanor Rathbone, who had persuaded Beveridge to join her Family Endowment Society whilst he was Director of the London School of Economics (LSE) in the 1920s and had introduced child allowances for LSE staff from 1925 onwards.

Eleanor Rathbone was one of the most truly independent Members of Parliament (MP) who ever sat in the House of Commons. The peculiar constituency which she represented from 1929 until her death on 2 January 1946 – the 'Combined Universi-ties' – favoured her unique reforming zeal and forthright political style. Few MPs have been so devoted to the principle of thorough research as the basis for social reform as Rathbone and few have been so determined to follow through the results of that research.

She is best known as the MP who, almost single-handed in the early days, led the campaign for family allowances. In fact, she began this work long before she became an MP. It was in the '1917 Club' in Gerrard Street, Soho (so-called after the February Revolution against the Czar of Russia) that she convened the first meeting of the 'Family Endowment Committee'. She had already contributed an article on the subject to the leading academic journal in economics, *The Economic Journal*, and she invited two young economics students, Emile Burns and Elinor Burns, to join her Committee, together with colleagues who had worked with her in her social research and in the campaign for women's suffrage, and a pro-suffrage journalist, Mr H.N. Brailsford.

They produced a one shilling pamphlet entitled *Equal Pay and the Family: A Proposal for the National Endowment of Motherhood* in 1918, using the example of the allowances paid to the wives of servicemen to reinforce her own argument based on the statistics of poverty and income distribution. Rathbone was familiar with these statistics, having worked for many years in the tradition of Charles Booth, with his surveys of poverty in London (1889–97), making detailed observations and collecting facts on the scale and nature of poverty in Liverpool in the decade before the First World War. This work had demonstrated the peculiar adverse effects of casual labour in the docks, at that time the biggest single source of employment in Liverpool. Her report, *How the Casual Labourer Lives*, was published in 1909 and was based on an investigation of family budgets collected and tabulated by a small committee (Stocks 1949: 62). She showed the connection between low wages and malnutrition among young children. It was followed by a similar painstaking study on *The Condition of Widows under the Poor Law in Liverpool*, published in 1913.

It was this tradition of thorough social and economic research which made it possible for Rathbone and her colleagues to produce such effective arguments for the reforms advocated in the booklet, *National Endowment of Motherhood*. However, Sidney Webb warned her that for any great social reform there was a time lag of about nineteen years between the dawn of an idea and its acceptance by public opinion (Stocks 1949: 86). In the case of family allowances the time lag from this first pamphlet to the Family Allowance Act of 1945 was twenty-seven years. All through this long period it was her main, although certainly not her only, preoccupation.

Rathbone herself was never a socialist and was indeed in 1931 briefly committed to the support of the National Government. However, even in that year on September 18th, when the Government proposed a 10 per cent cut in the unemployment benefits, her immediate reaction was to query whether it would not be better to increase taxation on higher incomes or luxury spending. Although she came from a wealthy family, her biographer Mary Stocks, comments that she always 'looked sympathetically on proposals which involved the redistribution of wealth through taxation and the elimination of wide discrepancies of material well-being between rich and poor' (Stocks 1949: 188).

This passion for social justice led her into increasingly bitter conflict with the next Conservative government of the mid-1930s, especially in relation to their treatment of the unemployed and their rejection of her arguments on child nutrition. She used the new findings of medical research on calories and vitamins to support the results of her earlier research on family budgets and cost of living.

It was of course mainly the Second World War which changed the climate of opinion on this and many other social reforms. This was true of the United States as well as Britain, although the New Deal already embraced some more egalitarian policies in the 1930s. Williamson and Lindert (1980), although they emphasise strongly the statistical problems, have no hesitation in character-ising the two world wars and the Civil War as periods of significant reduction in inequality. Social justice and social cohe-sion, neglected or rejected as wishy-washy liberal ideals before the Second World War in Britain, now became an essential element in sustaining civilian morale. Reformers like John Maynard Keynes and William Beveridge were once more invited to participate in the highest levels of policy-making. In June 1941, the British govern-ment appointed an inter-departmental Committee under the chairmanship of Beveridge to report on the whole problem of social insurance and allied services. The famous 'Beveridge Report' appeared in November 1942 and was based on three key assumptions:

1. the acceptance of family allowances
2. a comprehensive health service
3. full employment.

These were the three foundations of the post-war welfare state. Largely due to the persistent advocacy of Rathbone, the first of these principles now proved relatively uncontroversial and the Family Allowance Act went through in 1945. The 1945 Act was not all that Rathbone had campaigned for and she did not live to see the Welfare State flourish in the 1950s and 1960s in Britain and other countries, nor the beginnings of its decline in the 1980s and 1990s. Nor did she witness the widening gap between rich and poor, which has reversed the egalitarian trends of the 1940s and 1950s in Eastern as well as in Western Europe, in North as well as in South America, in China as well as in Japan. If she had seen it, it is unlikely in the extreme that she would have seen any connection between these trends and changes in technology, but that is the theme to which I turn in the second part of this chapter.

LONG WAVES AND TECHNOLOGY

Probably the most thorough, although certainly still controversial, studies of the long-term trends in the distribution of income and ownership of wealth in the United States are those of Williamson and Lindert (1980). They point out that already in the 1830s, in his classic study *Democracy in America*, Alexis de Tocqueville (1839), although very impressed by some egalitarian trends in US society, nevertheless suggested that industrialisation could lead to much greater inequality:

> I am of the opinion ... that the manufacturing aristocracy which is growing up under our eyes is one of the harshest that ever existed...the friends of democracy should keep their eyes anxiously fixed in this direction, for if a permanent inequality of conditions and aristocracy ... penetrates into America, it may be predicted that this is the gate by which they will enter.
>
> (de Tocqueville 1839/1963: 16)

This inspired intuitive observation by de Tocqueville became a definitive hypothesis in the classic paper of Simon Kuznets (1955), 'Economic growth and inequality', in which he suggested that growing inequality was characteristic of economies during the process of industrialisation, while 'mature' economies would be characterised by more egalitarian trends.

Williamson and Lindert (1980) argue that both in the United States and Britain the evidence supports the Kuznets hypothesis over the whole period of industrialisation, with growing inequality characteristic of both countries during most of the nineteenth century. In their painstaking research they deal with both the distribution of income and the ownership of wealth and argue that the two are closely related over the long term. Whilst they emphasise very strongly the poor quality and unreliability of the data on both incomes and wealth, especially in the period before the 1870s, they nevertheless feel able to make some tentative generalisations. In particular, they argue that the nature and direction of technical change during industrialisation favoured a persistent trend towards greater inequality. They place much greater emphasis on this than on social and fiscal policies but they do not pay much attention to the specifics of various waves of technology, nor to business cycles. They identify some periods of temporary reversal of the trend towards greater inequality, but they associate these periods (1800–20, 1860s, 1910s) primarily with the incidence of wars, with their strong demand for unskilled labour and their tendency to full employment.

Other US economists, such as Brian Berry et al (1994), argue that there have been other causes of the tendencies towards greater inequality in the United States:

> In the two-hundred year history of American macro-economic development there have been four great surges in inequality. Each followed a stagflation crisis and was accompanied by a turn of the electorate to more conserva-tive commercially-oriented candidates for the Presidency and Congress. Each surge was followed in turn by an egal-itarian backlash in which a political agenda dominated by technological innovation, efficiency and growth was replaced by one concerned with social innovation, equality and redistribution.
>
> (Berry et al 1994: Abstract)

Should these long swings be attributed simply to electoral pendulum-type changes in political mood over successive genera-tions or are they related in some way to changes in the economy and in technology?

At the simplest level, it is of course obvious that the standard of living for all of us depends on the achievements of science and technology. Since Adam Smith (1776/1974) the role of technical change in economic growth has been universally accepted by all schools of economists. The so-called 'new growth theory' gives to research, development and education a more central role than earlier growth models but no economist of repute had ever denied their importance. However, it is one thing to pay lip-service to the importance of science and technology in economic and social change but quite another thing to study this interdependent relationship in depth, i.e. to deploy the patient skills which Rathbone deployed in her studies of household budgets and apply them to the empirical study of the actual process of technical change in firms, in industries, in nations and in the world economy. In the first half of this century, almost the only economist to attempt this was Joseph Schumpeter and for this reason research on the economics and sociology of technical change is usually described as 'neo-Schumpeterian'. Its relevance to the problems of income distribution and social cohesion is especially evident in relation to the long cycles of investment behaviour and unemployment which he placed at the centre of his theory.

Schumpeter suggested in his *magnum opus* on *Business Cycles* (1939) that waves of new investment were generated by the diffusion of new technologies. In his theory, the ability and initiative of entrepreneurs, drawing upon the discoveries and ideas of scientists and inventors, create entirely new opportunities for investment, growth and employment. The exceptional profits made from these innovations are then the decisive signal to swarms of imitators generating band-wagon and multiplier effects throughout the system. Following the Russian economist, Nikolai Kondratieff, he argued that successive industrial revolutions led to long cycles of about 50 years' duration (see Table and Figure 8.1). Schumpeter studied the extraordinarily rapid growth of the cotton and iron industries in the first industrial revolution, of steam power and railways in the second and of electrification in the third. He observed that innovations tend to cluster together in relation to new infrastructures, so that the growth of the economy depends on a succession of industrial revolutions.

In a passage which is seldom referred to, Keynes (1930) fully acknowledged the significance of these influences on investment behaviour:

> In the case of fixed capital it is easy to understand why fluctuations should occur in the rate of investment. Entrepreneurs are induced to embark on the production of fixed capital or deterred from doing so by their expectations of the profits to be made. Apart from the many minor reasons why these should fluctuate in a changing world, Professor Schumpeter's explanation of the major movements may be unreservedly accepted.
>
> (Keynes 1930: 134)

Table 8.1 Long Waves

Kondratieff Wave	Cycle	Recession Trough of Depression	Core Inputs	Carrier Branches	Infrastructures
1st	1780s–1840s	1820s 1830s 1842–43	COTTON YARN IRON	Cotton textiles Other textiles Iron products	Ports Canals Water power Turnpike roads
2nd	1840s–1890s	1870s 1880s 1890s	COAL COAL GAS	Steam engines Railways Mechanisation Gas Machine tools	Iron – rail networks Telegraphy Steamships Gas light & heat
3rd	1890s–1940s	1920s 1930s 1930–34	STEEL	Electrification Electrical and heavy engineering Heavy chemicals Non-ferrous metals	Electric power Steel ships Global steel rail networks Telephones
4th	1940s–1990s	1970s 1980s 1990s	OIL NATURAL GAS	Automobiles Consumer durables Refineries Synthetic materials Automation	Motor highways Airlines Tankers Roll-on, roll-off
5th	1990s?– ?	?	MICRO-ELECTRONICS	Computers Video, telephone equipment software, info services	"Information highways" E-mail Air freight

A DIFFERENT SET OF TECHNOLOGIES
BEHIND EACH "GOLDEN AGE"

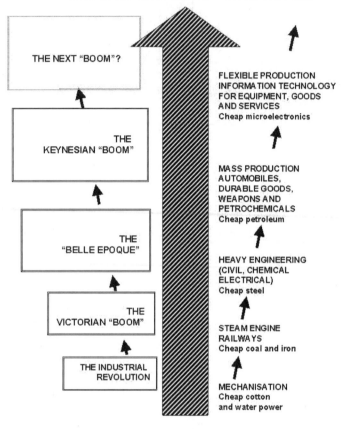

Source: C. PEREZ (1998)

Figure 8.1 Historical experience

The big investment booms and full employment of the 1850s and 1860s, or of the *belle époque* before the First World War, or of the 'Golden Age' of the 1950s and 1960s were followed by fairly prolonged periods of recession, depression and high unemployment. In Schumpeter's scheme, these recessions were the result of the erosion of profits from the previous wave of technology and the necessity for a new infrastructure and new industries to unleash the next wave. His theory is still controversial; opposition has

158

come both from more orthodox mainstream economists, who have been preoccupied with the shorter business cycles, and from orthodox Marxists, who drove Kondratieff to an early death in a Siberian labour camp in the 1930s.

In the 1920s, some US economists and businessmen had assumed that Henry Ford had superseded Karl Marx and that a bull market on the Stock Exchange could continue long into the future. In his *Short History of Financial Euphoria*, John Kenneth Galbraith (1993: 80) points out that just before the Wall Street crash of 1929, Irving Fisher and other US economists believed that stock prices were not over-valued and had reached a permanently high plateau. This neglect of both long and short business cycles was repeated in the 1990s when references were frequently made to the supposed 'end of history' and 'a new paradigm' of low inflation, full employment and high growth was supposed to have eliminated the business cycle. Alan Greenspan expressed some doubts about this but euphoria was widespread in the late 1990s.

If the test of a theory in the social sciences, as in the natural sciences, is its predictive power, then the ideas of Kondratieff and Schumpeter come out of this test in the twentieth century rather well. At a time when more orthodox Marxists were predicting the collapse of capitalism and its final crisis in the 1930s, Kondratieff had pointed to the possibility of a new capitalist growth boom. When the biggest-ever boom did in fact materialise in the 1950s and 1960s, long wave theorists such as Ernest Mandel pointed to the probability of a new deep recession. This was at a time when many economists and government advisers, such as those at the Organisation for Economic Cooperation and Development (OECD), assumed that the problem of mass unemployment would never return. Even in the 1970s, they continued to believe this despite the mounting evidence of structural unemployment (see, for example, the OECD McCracken Report 1977). In the 1930s, however, many economists had believed the opposite: that unemployment would remain at a permanently high level. Mainstream economics thus showed a persistent inability to understand or cope with the problems of mass unemployment and of structural change related to new technologies and with the problem of long swings in the world economy, whose very existence was denied.

Those economists and technologists who saw in computer technology, information technology and the Internet an enormous potential for new employment and a new wave of high investment and high growth were not mistaken. There is indeed such a potential but all previous experience shows that when a new pervasive technology enters the economic system, it can do so only after a prolonged social process of learning, reform and adaptation of old institutions. It was Carlota Perez (1983) who pointed out that there would be a mis-match between the institutions created to regulate the previously dominant technology and those needed to regulate a new one. The technical, political and economic uncertainties are so great that an uneven and conflict-ridden process is the rule rather than the exception. Temporary over-capacity in the fastest growing new industries was characteristic of all the big technologies in the past, as in semi-conductors and computers today. There was huge over-capacity in the Detroit automobile industry in the 1930s, and in the British cotton industry in the 1830s. No one can predict accurately at the time what will be the future size and characteristics of such new markets, still less the share of the individual firms or countries. These uncertainties are compounded by waves of euphoria and panic in the financial markets and by the general instability of investment in a capitalist market economy. The Internet bubble is no exception to this general rule, as the *Economist* magazine has forcefully pointed out on several occasions (1999).

GROWING INEQUALITY IN PERIODS OF STRUCTURAL ADJUSTMENT

Unemployment in periods of deep structural change is itself one of the main sources of inequality. These periods have been well described as 'crises of structural adjustment' because there is a mismatch between the skills and institutions of the older technologies and those which are needed for the new wave of technologies. Shortages and surpluses exist side by side as in the case of the shortage of software designers and engineers which persisted ever since the 1970s right through a period of massive unemployment. It was for this reason that Schumpeter maintained that aggregate statistics of GNP or of industrial production can conceal as much as they reveal since they are the outcome of diverse trends in the economy. There is general agreement that structural unemployment has been the main problem from the 1970s onwards, especially in Europe. However, although it has often been severe, unemployment has not been the only source of growing inequality

160

Table 8.2 General pattern of changes in the dispersion of earnings in the 1970s and 1980s. Hourly earnings or earnings of full-time workers

	1970s	1980s	Comments on extent and type of changes in dispersion
Australia	-	+	Increase in the dispersion from 1979 onwards
Austria	-	+	Increase from 1980 to 1989
Belgium		+	Slight increase due to gains at top over 1983-88
Canada	0	+	Increase mainly due to gains at top
Denmark		0	Slight gains at top and bottom
Finland	-	0	Slight gains at top and bottom
France	-	-/+	Decrease in dispersion ended in 1983
Germany	0	-	Decrease mainly due to gains at bottom
Italy	-	0	Gains at top and bottom
Japan		+	Increase due to gains at top
Netherlands	0	-/+	Slight decrease to 1984, then slight increase
Norway		0	Gains at top and bottom
Portugal		+	Increase between 1985 and 1990
Spain	--/0	+	Sharp decrease in mid-1970s, rise in 1980s
Sweden	0	0/+	Increase after 1986, except for low-paid women
United Kingdom	-	++	Increase from 1979 onwards
United States	+	++	Increase for men only in 1970s; strong gains at top in 1980s

Key: + Increase in dispersion
++ Strong increase
- Decrease
-- Strong decrease
0 No clear change (perhaps changes at top and bottom working in opposite directions)

over the last twenty years. Changes in earnings have also been a very important source of inequality (see Table 8.2).

As the notion of 'information-rich' and 'information-poor' households suggests, social inequality is not only a question of employment and unemployment. Each new wave of technical change brings with it many social benefits in the form of more new skilled occupations and professions, and higher standards of living for many people based on the growth of new industries and services. But each wave also brings high social costs in the form of erosion of old skills and occupations, the decline of some older industries, services and industrial areas. This uneven distribution of social costs and benefits occurs also on an international scale with some nations taking full advantage of the new technologies and others unable to do so. This international dimension is discussed in the fourth section of this chapter.

The effects of this uneven distribution of social costs and benefits are clearly visible in the statistics of earnings for the 1980s (see Table 8.2). Twelve of seventeen OECD countries showed an increased dispersion of earnings in the 1980s, four showed no change and only one (Germany) showed a decrease. In the 1970s the reverse was true. In that decade only one country showed an increase in inequality – the United States – while most others showed a decrease in dispersion. These statistics are for income before tax. Taking into account the fact that, as we have seen, fiscal changes in the UK and many other countries were regressive in this period, the increase of inequality in incomes has been substantial for those in employment as well as the unemployed.

Similar changes took place in previous waves of technical change: the earnings of engine drivers and fitters in the nineteenth century, of electricians in the 1890s, of assembly line workers in the 1940s and 1950s, and of software engineers and programmers in the 1980s, were all above the average earnings of the time. It is obvious that in any market system, the shortage of workers in rapidly expanding occupations will have these effects because of lags in supply. Consequently, periods of rapid structural change have generally been associated with increased inequality of incomes, arising both from increased dispersion of earnings and from high levels of unemployment.

The Secretary-General of the OECD, M. Paye, described the high levels of unemployment in the early 1990s as 'disturbing, perhaps alarming' and in the past the alarm bells which were ringing, whether in the 1830s, the 1880s or 1930s, ultimately led in Britain and elsewhere to programmes of social reform, educational reform, employment policies, and fiscal changes designed to mitigate the worst effects of these problems of structural change and to share the burdens more equally.

As we have seen, Berry et al (1994), following in the tradition of Kuznets, have suggested that income dispersion increased in the early stages of industrialisation and economic growth, diminishing with maturity. Berry et al proposed that alternating periods of wider and lesser dispersion corresponded to long (Kondratieff) cycles of economic development: 'It is in the immediate post stag-flation decade that inequality surges' (Berry et al 1994: 10). These surges of inequality in the 1830s, the 1880s, the 1920s and the 1980s were associated with the downturn of the long wave, with major structural changes, with demand for new skills (Williamson and Lindert, 1980) and high profits in new industries. The excep-tionally high profits from new technologies were obvious in the case of Microsoft in the 1980s and 1990s, of Ford in the 1920s, of Carnegie and the steel industry in the 1880s, of the railway magnate and speculator George Hudson in the 1840s, or of Arkwright and his water-frame cotton spinning in the 1790s.

Initially, strongly pro-business governments tend to aggravate the growing inequality, believing that a dose of strong medicine is needed to set the economy right, but ultimately, according to Berry et al's analysis, this leads to a political revulsion against the hard-ships which these policies incur (Jackson and the Homestead Act, etc. in the 1830s, the Anti-Trust Legislation and other reforms in the 1890s, and the New Deal etc., in the 1930s and 1940s).

Similar trends can be detected in social and political history in Britain and other countries as well as the US. The combined effect of prolonged periods of high unemployment together with the increased dispersion of earnings and increasing regressive taxation has been to create or to enlarge an 'underclass' in Britain, Russia, France, Spain and many other countries. A huge underclass already existed in Mexico, Brazil and most other countries of Latin America and Africa and this is growing now in Asia also. A rise in social tensions, crime and ethnic hostility was observable almost everywhere in the 1980s and was clearly associated with the loss of social cohesion and increasing insecurity of employment. The reduction in crime in the US in the 1990s was not simply due to new methods of policing but also to the temporarily lower levels of unemployment.

THE INTERNATIONAL DIMENSIONS OF INEQUALITY

The international dimension of the growth of inequality is even more serious than the domestic problems in the richer countries since the poverty in the third world is far more extreme. Since the industrial revolution and the huge changes in technology over the

Table 8.3 Estimates of trends in per capita GNP (1960 US$ and Prices, 1750–1977)

Year	Developed countries	Third World	Gaps
	(1) Per capita	(2) Per capita	(3) Ratio of the most developed to the least developed
1750	182	188	1.8
1800	198	188	1.8
1860	324	174	4.5
1913	662	192	10.4
1950	1054	203	17.9
1970	2229	380	25.7

Source: Bairoch 1981: 7–8

past two centuries, variations in country growth rates have been very wide. In particular, a group of countries, today referred to as 'developed' or 'industrialised' drew far ahead of the rest of the world (later known as 'under-developed') (see Table 8.3, Column 3).

Abramovitz (1986) coined the expression 'social capability' to describe that capacity to make institutional changes which led to this divergence in growth rates. He was himself one of the pioneers of 'growth accounting' but, as he pointed out, the accumulation of capital and increase in the labour force are not in themselves sufficient to explain these varying rates of economic growth. The huge divergence in growth rates which is so obvious a feature of long-term economic growth over the past two centuries must be attributed in large measure to the presence or absence of social capability for institutional change, and especially for those types of institutional change which facilitate and stimulate a high rate of technical change, i.e. innovation systems. Institutional changes were, of course, essential for the accumulation of capital itself.

The rise of pervasive new technologies involves the emergence of some qualitatively new features in the social and economic system. Partly as a result of historical accidents and partly as a result of deliberate policies, their domination of international institutions and naval power, some countries proved more adept in exploiting the potential of these new technologies both in world trade and in domestic growth. Many other countries were able to catch up with the leaders by a combination of imitation and autonomous innovation. Until the 1990s, some of the East Asian countries were good

Table 8.4 Comparative growth rates sub-continental regions 1965–99

GDP % p.a.	1965–1980	1980–1989	1990–999 (est)
East Asia	7.5	7.9	7.2
South Asia	3.9	5.1	5.5
Africa (sub-Sahara)	4.0	2.1	2.7
Latin America	5.8	1.6	3.1
GDP per Capita % p.a.	1965–1980	1980–1989	1990–1999 (est)
East Asia	5.0	6.3	5.7
South Asia	1.5	2.9	3.4
Africa (sub-Sahara)	1.1	−1.2	0.2
Latin America	3.5	−0.5	1.2

Source: World Bank Development Report 1991; Own estimates 1990s

examples of accelerated catch-up. Both their rapid catch-up in the 1970s and 1980s and the crisis which they experienced in the mid-1990s demand some explanation in terms of technical and institutional change.

Whereas real per capita incomes were actually falling during the 1980s in Africa and Latin America, they were rising quite fast in south Asia and very rapidly in east Asia (see Tables 8.4 and 8.5). The east Asian countries were especially successful in expanding their production and exports of electronics and telecommunication equipment, which were by far the fastest growing in world trade. Although they are all relatively new, the electronic industries vary in their skill intensity and technology intensity. The general pattern is clearly for the most skill- and technology-intensive activities to remain in Japan with the least skill-intensive increasingly based in the second tier of south-east Asian countries or even in south Asia. The 'Four Tigers' and China occupy an intermediate position but analysis of the trends in their exports shows a steadily rising ratio of skill-intensive and technology-intensive products. This shift was made possible by active education, industrial and technology policies within these countries (Amsden 1991, 1992; Amsden and Hikino 1991; Wade 1990).

What the post-war experience demonstrates therefore is an extremely uneven process of catch-up by developing countries, depending upon their technical capability and on imports of technologies. But the import of technologies is very far from the costless diffusion of 'information' assumed in some versions of

Table 8.5 Distribution of developing countries by rates of growth of GDP
per capita 1960–84 (number of countries)

Growth of GDP/Capita	1960–69	1970–74	1975–79	1980–84
2 per cent and above				
Latin America	19	17	15	1
Sub-Saharan Africa	25	18	16	5
South Asia	2	1	5	4
East Asia	7	9	7	6
0.1–1.9 per cent				
Latin America	5	8	6	1
Sub-Saharan Africa	10	13	6	7
South Asia	3	1	2	3
East Asia	3	–	–	1
0 per cent and below				
Latin America	2	1	5	24
Sub-Saharan Africa	12	16	25	35
South Asia	2	5	–	–
East Asia	–	1	3	3

Source: UNCTAD (1986) *Trade and Development Report, 1986*, New York:
United Nations

economic theory. Technologies cannot be taken 'off the shelf' and simply put into use anywhere. Without infrastructural investment in education, training, research and development (R&D) and other scientific and technical activities, very little can be accomplished by way of assimilation of imported technologies. The Asian countries were by far the most active in promoting these policies. Michael Hobday (1995) has pointed to the variety of strategies in the east Asian countries, all designed in different ways steadily to upgrade local technological capability. The contrast between the rapid rise in the performance of in-house R&D in firms in both south Korea and Taiwan, and its low level, stagnation or non-existence in firms in most developing countries is especially notable.

The rise of in-house R&D in the 1970s led to an extraordinary increase in numbers of patents, and this is perhaps the most striking confirmation of the active learning system in South Korea and Taiwan. Between 1963–85 and 1997–8, the average number of patents taken out per annum in the USA by Brazil, Argentina and Mexico together increased from ninety-four per annum to 163 per annum, but in the same period, the numbers taken out by the three Asian Tigers increased from thirty-six per annum to over 5,000 per annum (see Table 8.6). The figures for 1997–8 were not

Table 8.6 Patents granted in the United States to owners in various
countries, average numbers per annum in various periods
1963–98

Country	1963–1985	1983–1989	1990–1996	1997–1998
Taiwan	26	327	1,577	2,578
S. Korea	8	83	853	2,575
Singapore	2	9	48	107
Mexico	54	41	45	51
Brazil	18	30	59	68
Argentina	22	19	28	44
Total all countries	64,391	80,820	110,418	129,752

Source: Kumar (1997) based on data from US Patents and Trademarks Office
(1997) for Columns 2 and 3; TAF Report from US Patent Office (1999)
for Columns 1 and 4.

yet affected by the downturn in the Asian economies in that period
because of the lag in the patent series based on grant of patent in
the US Patent Office.

Firms in both Korea and Taiwan were so successful in their
catch-up that they began to export technology themselves and to
invest overseas in older industrial countries like Britain as well as
in the less developed countries of south-east Asia. However,
despite their great success in the 1970s and 1980s and indeed,
partly because of it, the global economy in the 1990s presented
new and acute problems for those catch-up countries which made
good progress in closing the gap in manufacturing. The liberalisation of capital movements which had taken place exposed all
countries to the instability and shocks which occur in any part of
the system. Events during 1997 and 1998 showed that these shocks
can be propagated throughout the system and that however well
the national economy is performing, it is always still part of a
broader global economic and political system.

Many of the comments on the east Asian crisis of 1997–8 are
characterised by emphasis on the supposed sins of the Asian
governments. In particular, they have blamed corruption of
governments for some of the unwise and inept investment decisions
of the 1990s. Of course, there has been corruption in many Asian
countries and in some, especially Indonesia, it has been on a very
large scale. There has also been corruption in European countries
and in the US. But it is fanciful to put the whole blame for the
collapse on corruption and to ignore the misallocation of private

investment. As Jeffrey Sachs has written in the *International Herald Tribune*:

> It is somehow comforting, as in a good morality tale, to blame corruption and mismanagement in Asia for the crisis. Yes, these exist, and they weaken economic life. But the crisis itself is more pedestrian. No economy can easily weather a panicked withdrawal of confidence, especially if the money was flooding in just months before...
>
> The problems emerged in the private sector. In all of the countries, international money-market managers and investment banks went on a lending binge from 1993 to 1996. To a varying extent in all of the countries, the short-term borrowing from abroad was used, unwisely, to support longterm investments in real estate and other non-exporting sectors.

(Sachs 1997)

The problems of catch-up in technology will now be aggravated by the social tensions engendered by the investment crisis and the International Monetary Fund (IMF) medicine. In a region previously characterised by rather high levels of employment and a strong demand for labour, unemployment became a serious social problem. The president of the World Bank, James Wolfensohn, was one of the first to recognise that the social problems associated with high unemployment would now require major policy attention, including World Bank programmes:

> The region must tackle social issues if it is to foster sustainable economic recovery and East Asia's financial crisis risks undermining one of the most remarkable economic and social achievements of modern history. What began as a financial crisis has spilled over into the real economy, severely hitting both production and employment.
>
> In that case, was the miracle a mirage? Emphatically not. No other group of countries in the world has produced more rapid economic growth and dramatic reductions in poverty...
>
> They did it by getting the fundamentals right – with high savings, a commitment to education, sound fiscal policies

and an outward orientation. But as the crisis has revealed, political, financial and corporate structures were not well suited to cope with the demands of an increasingly globalised economy.

(Wolfensohn 1998)

As recent events have shown, dependence on the global economy, and on the IMF and World Bank, can be a mixed blessing so that the reform of the IMF is now becoming an urgent question for the management of the global economy. Again, as Sachs (1998) has pointed out, the lack of accountability and transparency in the operations of the IMF means that disagreement with its advice is now often regarded as synonymous with a sinful rejection of financial rectitude punishable by the markets. Yet its advice has often been mistaken, and not only in east Asia. It forecast growth of 1.5 per cent in Mexico in 1995 after the Mexican financial crisis, but actual growth was minus 6.1 per cent, and again in Argentina forecast growth was 2 per cent and actual growth minus 4.6 per cent. Its handling of successive crises in Latin America in 1995, in Bulgaria in 1996 and east Asia in 1997 and 1998 calls into question its ability to handle the volatility of the private capital market in a way which does not damage future growth in countries in which the 'fundamentals' for sustained growth are relatively favourable.

CONCLUSIONS

Cycles of over-capacity and of shortages are a familiar accompaniment of waves of technical change. The over-capacity in Asia in electronic consumer goods was one such episode and the over-capacity in memory chips and semi-conductors was another; the Bank for International Settlements (BIS) pointed to these problems in successive Annual Reports:

[I]ndications of excessive investment in particular sectors had already emerged in 1996. In that year, the massive investment in Asia's electronic industry contributed to conditions of oversupply and a resulting price collapse in world markets. But investment has sharply increased in other areas as well (such as automobile construction, household appliances and electricity generation) at the risk

of flooding local and foreign markets ... Overinvestment
in particular sectors has tended to erode the rates of return
on capital in recent years.

(BIS 1998: 36)

These phenomena in the 'real' economy interact with political
events and with financial markets to generate the instability characteristic of the periods of structural 'crises of adjustment'. In the
1890s as in the 1990s, outward flows of speculative investment to
'emerging economies' aggravated this instability. The headlong deregulation and liberalisation of capital movements in the 1970s
and 1980s has created a particularly unstable situation in the
world economy at the turn of the millennium, as both the speed
and scale of capital movements are greatly increased by the use of
information technology and of ingenious financial innovations
such as derivatives. The mathematical pretensions of the derivatives models which underlie the speculative investments of the
'hedging funds', even if they are developed by Nobel prize-winners,
would be laughable if they were not tragic in their consequences.

The present phase of the 'information revolution' therefore calls
out more than ever for institutional and social innovations which
could create a stable regulatory framework for the constructive
application of this extraordinary powerful technology in world-
wide economic growth. Another *belle époque* in which the potential productivity gains of information technology are more fully
realised is by no means inevitable. It depends on the policies which
are now adopted.

It is not possible here to prescribe a detailed set of policy
proposals but what can be done in conclusion is to indicate the
main directions in which future policies should move, first of all to
mitigate the worst effects of the present crisis and later, to shape a
more stable social environment for the world economy.

Firstly, as many economists and politicians have now recognised, the IMF and World Bank should be reformed to bring them
closer to the original Keynesian ideal. They need the resources and
the mode of governance to enable them to prevent temporary
problems of particular countries from degenerating into general
deflationary recessions.

Secondly, as Wolfensohn, president of the World Bank, has
indicated, social policies should assume a much higher priority.
The general trend of these policies should be designed to reduce
inequalities in the system, both at the national and the

international level. World-wide redistributive policies should be financed by the 'Tobin Tax', a tax on the speculative transactions in international financial markets, first proposed by James Tobin. This would not only provide much-needed additional finance for international institutions but would also help to reduce the huge surges of short-term capital movements which destabilise governments and societies.

Thirdly, these movements should in any case be far more closely regulated and controlled, as for example, by the tax on short-term capital transactions imposed in Chile.

Finally, the trend towards inegalitarian taxation and social policies should be reversed by a return to the principles of redistribution, as advocated by most leading economists since John Stuart Mill and as so energetically pursued by idealistic social reformers, such as Rathbone and Mill himself. Movements in these directions might seem a distant and even utopian ideal in the immediate future but in the light of the long-term changes discussed in this chapter, they may not be so remote and may be already important early in the twenty-first century.

9

INEQUALITY, WORK AND TECHNOLOGY IN THE SERVICES SECTOR

Gavin Poynter and Alvaro de Miranda

THE TRANSFORMATION OF WORK IN 'POST-INDUSTRIAL' SOCIETIES

Several authors have argued that recent decades have seen the end of industrialism and the birth of a new kind of post-industrial or post-modern society (Bell 1973, 1980; Toffler 1981; Naisbitt 1984; Pakulski and Waters 1996). The end of industrialism has been associated with the relative decline of manual employment and the traditional manufacturing or 'smoke-stack' industries that produce tangible goods. Post-industrial society has arisen with the emergence of new industries based upon the creation and manipulation of information and knowledge, or 'non-tangible' goods, and a vast expansion of the service sector. The growth of these industries is linked to a rise in non-manual occupations, the expansion of employment opportunities for women workers and the coming of what some have called the 'information' or 'network' age (Hamel and Prahalad 1996; Castells 1996).

Enthusiasts of the transformation thesis have come from the academic and business worlds (Bell 1980; Masuda 1985; Drucker 1986; Stonier 1983; Hamal and Prahalad 1996). At the centre of their argument is the role played by information and communication technologies (ICTs) in bringing about the transformation of work. The transformation, according to such optimists as Stonier, for example, leads to everyone becoming:

an aristocrat, a philosopher. A massively expanded education system to provide not only training and information
on how to make a living, but also on how to live. In late
industrial society we stopped worrying about food. In late
communicative society we will stop worrying about all
material resources.

(Stonier 1983:214)

The new world envisaged by the enthusiasts of the information age
is one in which the advanced industrial nations are freed from the
problem of economic scarcity and their workers are, in turn, freed
from routine and mundane tasks. According to this view, change in
the way that people work is accompanied by change in the organisational structures of the enterprises in which they are employed.
The old hierarchical form of management organisation, appropriate to the period of the dominance of the large scale factory, is
displaced by flatter, smaller units in which people work in teams
and are connected together through webs or networks. Traditional
management approaches that sought to command and control are
displaced by ones that emphasise co-ordination and commitment
and the knowledge workers of the future will be, 'selected,
rewarded and promoted according to competencies, values and
performance rather than seniority, formal skill or rate for the job'
(Warhurst and Thompson 1998: 3).

The optimists' view of the transformation of work which accom-
panies the emergence of the Information Age associates the new
ways of working with the end of work practices and forms of
industrial organisation that gave rise to alienation and inequality in
the workplace (Depres and Hiltrop 1995). The transformation of
work is synonymous with its democratisation and the provision of
opportunities for the majority of employees – regardless of gender,
race or social background – to achieve their potential and earn the
rewards that their educational attainments deserve.

This chapter critically assesses this optimistic perspective. It
focuses on the changes in work and the experience of work for
those employed in the service economy – the sector that has experienced rapid employment growth in recent years and the one in
which significant technological changes have occurred. The
chapter is designed to explain some of the key themes and issues
that arise for those who wish to get beyond the sweeping
pronouncements of the millennial kind and embark upon a critical
examination of the relationship between inequality and change at

work in the new century. There are many different dimensions to the experience of inequality at work. This chapter focuses on three themes which recur in the literature associated with the optimistic view of the future. This view perceives the future trajectory of work as taking a 'high road' toward a high skill, high wage economy (Milkman 1998). First, it is claimed by the optimists that recent changes in work have created the potential for a significant reduction in the number of boring and monotonous jobs that arose in the past in the typical manufacturing workplace in which the assembly line symbolised the 'degradation' of work (Zuboff 1988; Handy 1995). Second, optimists claim that rapid technological change has given rise to a process of up-skilling of staff who are increasingly finding themselves employed by enterprises that have become learning institutions (Gallie 1996: 142–4) and, finally, the optimists proclaim that the 'feminisation' of the workforce has led to changes in attitudes toward work and given rise to significant improvements in career prospects for women workers (Hirschhorn 1984). These themes are explored through the evidence provided by one important service sector, the financial services. Such a specific focus cannot give rise to conclusions that may be valid for the service sector as a whole but, in providing insights into developments at industry and workplace levels, it is hoped that the chapter raises questions and issues that may be useful to those who wish to examine changes at work in other service industries.

The chapter is divided into three parts. Part 1 outlines some of the challenges and difficulties faced in defining service industries, particularly in contemporary advanced economies where rapid technological change contributes to the blurring of industrial boundaries. It also briefly examines the ways in which technological change has contributed to developments in the organisation of work and the social and technical divisions of labour in these industries. Technological change provides opportunities for the re-shaping of work and the re-ordering of social relations within the workplace. Opportunities arise for traditional hierarchies to be challenged and new forms of work organisation to emerge. The new forms of work organisation may replicate previous patterns of inequality between employees or facilitate the emergence of new opportunities for career advancement for those staff previously confined to less skilled, low paid 'dead-end' jobs.

The rapid growth in employment in financial services in the 1960s and 1970s saw women's employment grow faster than men's. Typically, women took over clerical work, particularly cashier roles, from men. The work of the cashier was accorded a lower status as men were appointed to career positions that also carried with them substantial contractual advantages like cheap home and other loans and pensions. Male staff, on the career path, tended to stay with the company moving eventually into middle and senior administrative and management posts. The employment contracts for the majority of women staff precluded such progression. The profile of Barclays Bank staff in 1983 illustrates this gender divide. Of a total of 67,500 employees, two-thirds were women and more than three-fifths of these were in the bottom two grades (BIFU 1984: 3). Gender inequality in the financial services was embedded in the divide between low paid clerical functions carried out by women on the one hand and career oriented administrative and managerial positions held by men on the other. The rapid expansion of the financial services was facilitated by the reshaping of the technical division of labour – the feminisation of clerical work – and the reshaping of the social division of labour – the confinement of the vast majority of women to employment contracts that offered lower paid, lower valued and less skilled jobs (Crompton and Jones 1984). The restructuring of the financial services sector in the 1990s provided opportunities to challenge the inequalities that shaped the technical and social divisions of labour that emerged in the 1960s and 1970s. Before exploring whether enterprises seized this opportunity, it is necessary to briefly outline what is meant by the division of labour and explain how this is affected by the current changes occurring within the service sector.

At first sight the division of labour appears to be a straightforward concept. It is not. The technical division of labour refers to the division of tasks, skills and jobs found within a workplace or enterprise. People specialise in particular work functions. This is particularly true of an industrial society where the complex range of tasks required to produce goods or provide services are more than a single person can cope with. It is far more efficient for people to specialise. The divisions of labour that result are shaped by the 'technical' requirements or complexities of the product being made or service being provided. The social division of labour refers to the wider societal organisation of production and service provision. Here firms and enterprises exchange their products (finished or intermediate goods and services) with each other and employers exchange money (in the form of wages) to secure the labour power required to undertake work on their behalf. In capitalist society this exchange is regulated by product and labour markets. It is the role of these markets in regulating exchange between enterprises and between employers and workers that gives this dimension of the division of labour its specific social content and capitalist society its distinctive character. In practice, the parameters of the technical and social divisions of labour change with developments in technology and in accordance with the inter-actions between workers and managers. Managers usually super-vise work. In broad terms, they ensure that the technical division of labour within a workplace operates efficiently. The expansion of the management role in the twentieth century enterprise, in turn, has given rise to what is called the hierarchical division of labour within a workplace, a division that, put simply, refers to the distinction between the workers who do the work and those who supervise them (Sayer and Walker 1992: 15–20).

Part 2 provides evidence from the financial services sector to illustrate the complex changes that have occurred in enterprise and work organisation. Part 2 also explores how these developments have impacted on technical and social divisions of labour, the workforce and their experience of service work. In particular, the analysis focuses on the recent emergence of a new kind of work-place, the telecentre or call centre, a form of work organisation that has rapidly diffused across many service industries and one that has typically involved the employment of women workers (Fincham et al 1994). Finally, in Part 3, some tentative conclusions are drawn about the changing experience of work and an evalua-tion is made of the optimistic view presented by those who believe we are moving into a more egalitarian information age or 'compu-topia' (Masuda 1985).

DEFINING SERVICES

New ideas and values and new forms of work organisation have entered most workplaces over recent years. A new language has emerged in which employees are 'human resources', managers are 'facilitators' and 'enablers' and all service users are 'customers'. This customer orientation has spread to most areas of public life. As more and more employees consider themselves as service providers so it appears that all forms of employment are involved in some kind of service work. In short, it has become increasingly difficult in the advanced economies of countries like the US and Britain, to distinguish precisely what is a service sector enterprise and what is 'service' work. This confusion is reflected in the academic and business literature. The definition of services is a contested issue.

Historically, the definition of services arose from an analysis of capitalist development that was presented as a process of linear progression. The trajectory of industrial development was based upon sectoral change in which employment shifted in the advanced economies from a primary sector (agriculture) to a secondary sector (manufacturing) and then on to a tertiary or service sector. This thesis was first advanced by Fisher (1939) and Clark (1940). The thesis defined manufacturing as the making of tangible goods and commodities whilst services were associated with the provision of the intangible or non-material. The thesis was subsequently re-worked in the post-1945 period by authors like Bell (1973; 1980) for whom the shift to what he called a post-industrial society was characterised by the substitution of goods producing activities by those concerned with the provision of services. In his earlier writings Bell's argument concerning the emergence of post-industrial society rested mainly on the growth in new types of technical, scientific and professional occupations. By 1980 the advances in information technology enabled him to add the information dimension so that the concept of the post-industrial could be reworked into a theory of the information age. The new age was founded upon the convergence of the computing, electronic and telecommunications industries which transformed the social and cultural spheres as well as the techno-economic base (Kumar 1995: 13). For Bell, and other protagonists of the new age, the emergence of a vast number of workers whose main task was the use and manipulation of information and knowledge provided compelling evidence of the transition. For such authors the old nineteenth century preoccupation with labour as the main source of value in an economy was surpassed by the proposition that knowledge was the new source of value. The missionary zeal found in the writings of such authors as Bell (1973) and Toffler (1981) for the new information age has tended to distort the understanding and analysis of services industries in contemporary societies like the USA and Britain. This distortion has four main dimensions.

First, the growth in service sector employment was perceived by the enthusiasts of the information age from a north American and north European perspective which tended to ignore the growth of production industries and manufacturing employment in other regions of the world. From a global viewpoint, manufacturing production shifted location rather than experiencing significant decline and unleashed in the last decades of the twentieth century a new pattern of uneven capitalist development on a global scale (Henderson 1989; Dicken 1992). Second, employment growth in manufacturing industries has been overstated as an indicator of the development of industrial capitalism and, conversely, its relative decline has been overstated as evidence of its demise. Taking a longer term perspective, and presenting manufacturing employment in a relative context, a different picture emerges. In the US, for example, even during the period of rapid industrial expansion in the late nineteenth century, manufacturing employment stood at only 27 per cent of total employment. A century later, in 1989, the percentage of the total labour force employed in manufacturing had declined by a mere one per cent to 26 per cent. A similar picture of relative stability in manufacturing's share of the total labour force emerges for other nations like the Netherlands, Germany and Japan (Maddison 1991: 31). From this longer term perspective, a more important indicator of the continued importance of manufacturing industries has been their growth in output. This has maintained an albeit modest upwards trajectory even in those economies such as the UK, where the employment share of manufacturing has experienced a relatively sharper rate of decline than other advanced nations in Europe. This continued upward trend in output growth relative to employment has merely indicated the capacity of manufacturing industries, with the exception of brief periods of deep recession, to produce more using less labour, a phenomenon that Massey and others have referred to as 'jobless growth' (Massey 1988: 54).

A third distortion arose from the characterisation of the role of knowledge in the contemporary workplace. The diffusion of ICTs enhanced the knowledge base of existing work, leading to an upgrading of its content and value for the enterprise (Kumar 1995: 23), and also generated a significant rise in the number of knowledge workers employed. Simultaneously, ICTs improved the quality of work content and facilitated the expansion in the proportion of knowledge-based occupations. In practice, however, the evidence to support such claims is, at best, mixed. Employment in business services, for example, has significantly expanded over recent years. Business services include those occupations concerned with 'high tech' consultancy and the provision of advice on developing management information systems – often highly paid tasks undertaken by 'partners' employed in consultancy firms. However, business services also includes, companies who provide dedicated data and information processing services to manufacturing and service sector firms. Typically, such work involves data inputting and processing – highly mechanised and routinised tasks that demand little knowledge-input from employees whose numbers constitute a significant proportion of those employed in the business services sector. Put simply, working with information and data is not automatically synonymous with an upgrading of the knowledge content of many occupations. Paradoxically, the exponential growth in the production of electronic information and data may lead to a reduction in the proportion of non-manual occupations that are knowledge-based or require the exercise of tacit knowledge and individual discretion. Post-industrial and information society theorists accorded service work many virtuous characteristics that much of it did not deserve. Those who processed and utilised information were attributed with skills and knowledge that did not match their experience of work (Robins and Webster 1987; 1989; Webster 1995).

Finally, many information workers may not be directly involved on the shopfloor in making products like cars or other electrical consumer goods but may, nevertheless, provide essential components or intermediate goods that indirectly contribute to the process of production. In this sense, many software designers, programmers and information/database handlers, all relatively new occupations, provide 'intermediate' goods that are essential to the production of commodities but they have been erroneously given the status of providers of business services by official government publications, academics and business writers who, consciously or otherwise, through their categorisation of employment, consign industrial society to the history books. This distorted picture of developments that have taken place in contemporary advanced industrial societies tends to over-simplify the complex changes that have occurred in the social and technical divisions of labour in these economies. These changes have given rise to a significant growth in indirect labour and post-production activities like sales and marketing (Sayer and Walker 1992) and have created an increasingly complex inter-dependence between manufacturing and service industries in the contemporary world.

Whilst the argument presented so far questions the end of industrialism thesis, it would be wrong to conclude that little has changed. The increased complexity of the contemporary technical and social divisions of labour and the growth, for example, of service sector employment are observable everywhere in countries like the UK. The use of credit cards, the integration of telephonic and computer technologies, the emergence of the Internet as a business tool and the increasing importance of a wide range of other technological innovations have transformed the relationships between workplace, high street and home over recent years. These product and process innovations took off in the 1980s and realised a significant expansion of employment in many service industries including retail banking.

The financial services sector was, in many ways, the beneficiary of these developments in the 1980s but it also became their 'victim' in the 1990s. The expansion and increased complexity of the hierarchical and social divisions of labour had also generated a rise in operating costs and concerns about productivity levels in the service sector (Quinn and Gagnon 1985; Hammer 1990). The consequence of this was that the economic recession of the late 1980s and early 1990s, which impacted first on countries like the USA and UK, saw the first real attempt by many service sector enterprises to curtail employment growth, improve productivity and re-engineer work processes (Head 1996). The service sector that was to provide the base, according to many enthusiasts, of the emergence of a new information age was itself subjected to an uneven process of rationalisation and restructuring. 'Downsizing' and 'de-layering' flattened the hierarchical division of labour and re-engineering was adopted to reconfigure the social and technical divisions of labour within and between service sector enterprises and their counterparts in other spheres of the national and global economies.

It is this restructuring process that provides the context for an evaluation of the relationship between the service economy, technological innovation and inequality in the late 1990s. Traditional hierarchical patterns of work organisation in the financial services, particularly in the small high street branch, tended to provide career paths that favoured the male worker whilst the vast majority of women staff were confined to lower grades and non-managerial posts. The restructuring of work within the sector, facilitated by extensive investment in new technologies, provided new opportunities to address the inequalities between men and women in relation to skills development and career progression. In short, financial services provide a useful test of the optimists' view that contemporary technological and organisational change generates a significant shift toward a less hierarchical workplace in which the traditional patterns of gender inequality are removed.

RESTRUCTURING IN FINANCIAL SERVICES

During the 1980s and 1990s the financial services sector was the highest investor in information technologies within the UK (Rajan 1984; Fincham et al 1994). In the 1980s technological change took place within a highly conservative organisational and managerial context. By the late 1980s and early 1990s, many financial services companies recognised the necessity for organisational reform to accompany technical innovation. In general terms, retail banking took the lead in organisational and technological innovation and insurance companies and building societies followed. In the 1980s it was possible to identify different segments of the financial services sector. There were four main components – building societies, the insurance industry, the credit card industry and the banking industry. Banking was the largest employer within the sector and there was a clear institutional and functional distinction between the constituent parts. By the mid-1990s the sectoral and institutional distinctions began to break down and companies that had previously upheld the virtues of tradition and conservatism began to engage in a process of radical restructuring. There were four main catalysts of this transformation.

First, significant changes took place in the market conditions prevailing in financial services in the decade commencing in the latter part of the 1980s. The economic recession of 1989–92 impacted significantly on profit margins in all the main financial services industries. Banks were required to cover rising debt burdens whilst insurance companies were forced to meet a significant growth in claims from corporate and personal customers.

Second, changing market conditions were closely linked with changes in the structure of the financial services in countries like the UK. Deregulation in the mid-1980s sharpened competition between banks, building societies and insurance companies. Deregulation allowed companies to cross the traditional institutional divides and compete with one another in presenting new combinations of financial services to personal and corporate customers. The key task was to establish market share and a strong customer base through which the cross-selling of financial products could take place. This development led, in turn, to financial institutions concluding partnership arrangements with retail food stores and other organisations in order to exploit the opportunities presented by their customer-base. In this sense, deregulation facilitated the opening of financial services provision with, as a result, the development of what might be called 'blurred' boundaries between financial services and other industrial sectors as non-financial services companies like Tesco, Asda and Marks and Spencer began to offer either their own financial services packages or packages created through partnerships with banks and insurance institutions.

Third, financial services was a major investor in new technologies. In the 1960s and 1970s technical innovation had been largely used to support traditional branch structures of banks, building societies and insurance companies. Mainframe computers provided the processing power required to ease the burden on branch-based back office functions. Computerisation led to the centralisation of administrative tasks within processing centres miles away from the branch office. By the mid-1970s financial institutions began to establish on-line links between central mainframe databases and local branch offices. By the end of the 1970s and into the early 1980s computerisation spread to most workplaces within the sector and was no longer largely the preserve of the processing centre. The introduction of personal computers (PCs) and developments in digital communications technologies helped companies move towards an integration of their computer systems and enabled the introduction of automated teller machines (ATM) and electronic funds transfer at the point of sale (EFTPOS). These developments provided the opportunity for financial institutions to reconsider the relationship between 'back' and 'front' office functions. Technological advances facilitated organisational change whilst economic recession and sharpening competition demanded it. The 1990s witnessed a process of innovation that saw technologies used to break-up traditional patterns of work organisation rather than replicate them. A significant restructuring of work organisation and service delivery took place with many front office functions being transferred to regional customer service centres. Whereas technological change in 1980s had relatively little impact upon employment growth in areas like retail banking, in the 1990s it was utilised to implement rationalisation programmes in the leading UK retail banks. In the big four retail banks in the UK (HSBC/Midland, Natwest, Lloyds/TSB and Barclays) a reduction in the total number of employees was accompanied by an expansion in part-time, fixed contract and more casual forms of employment. Part-time employment was used as an instrument to control costs (Gregory and O'Reilly 1996).

Rationalisation and technical innovation in areas like retail banking was accompanied by a fourth catalyst of change – the concern amongst financial services institutions to raise productivity and efficiency and thus reduce their operating cost/income ratio. In broad terms, many institutions decided to focus primarily on their 'core' financial services activities, their financial services product portfolio, and outsource their non-core functions such as data processing and facilities management. This development enabled the expansion of the data processing industry and brought with it new contractual relations with service providers who were often companies, like Unisys, whose origins were in the computing industry. Changes in the technical and social divisions of labour within the financial services sector gave rise to an uneven process of restructuring. Employment levels in the main retail banking institutions declined. Across the sector as a whole, however, the expansion of financial services provision and the disaggregation of financial services into the 'wider external economy' created an overall increase in employment (Cressey and Scott 1992: 89).

Having identified the main catalysts of restructuring within financial services, it is now possible to examine their implications for work and the experience of work at the enterprise level. In particular the next section focuses on a relatively new and expanding area of service sector employment – the telecentre or call centre. The telecentre symbolises several of the themes of this chapter. Its development has arisen from the integration of advanced computer and telecommunications technologies and the utilisation of new software and distributed database systems. These have created opportunities for new forms of 'virtual' customer services to be delivered via the telephone and the Internet.

The process of technological change has facilitated significant organisational innovation within sectors like the financial services. Unencumbered by costly high street branch networks, non-financial institutions have entered the market place selling 'direct' a range of financial service products, including, for example, credit/debit cards and motor, household and other general insurance. The telecentres that deal with customer inquiries and the direct selling of products have typically been established as 'greenfield' sites – new buildings, purpose-built and located on newly constructed business parks or industrial estates. The workers employed in such centres have been mainly women whose employment conditions are very different from those that traditionally prevailed in the financial services sector.

The telecentre provides a cutting edge example of how technological change has contributed to the emergence of a form of work organisation in which the human/computer interface is the essence of a new type of customer-oriented service provision. The telecentre offers, therefore, a useful test of the optimists' claim that the advanced technologies of the information age facilitate the emergence of workplaces which remove the mundane and repetitive forms of manual labour associated with large scale factory production and enable the emergence of a more egalitarian workplace in which the creation, processing and analysis of data is a central function.

THE TELECENTRE – A POST-INDUSTRIAL WORKPLACE?

Telecentres (or call centres) consist of workplaces in which customer service telephone agents are physically co-located in one large room or building. The agents are supported by sophisticated information and communication technology systems which assist them to answer telephone enquiries from customers and/or undertake sales and marketing activities (telesales or telemarketing). Telecentres vary in size from a few to a few hundred seats. They often provide a twenty-four hour service and are staffed on flexible shift systems by full- and part-time employees. Large national and international organisations often have their own telecentres. Telecentre functions are also outsourced to specialist telecentre providers servicing more than one organisation. Outsourcing is particularly favoured by enterprises that do not have a sufficient volume of telephone business to justify their own 24-hour telecentre operation, but some large organisations also prefer this method of operation. For example, SITEL Corporation of the US established six telecentre sites in the UK in the 1990s and provide services for such clients as the National Health Service, British Gas, Shell, Volkswagen, Nissan and Disneyland, Paris. SITEL's revenue from these operations was £77 million in 1997 and was projected to rise to £250 million by 2002. This form of outsourcing of telecentre operations was projected to expand within Europe by 20–25 per cent in 1998 (Payne 1998).

184

Telecentre Growth

The number of telecentres has expanded dramatically. The US and Europe have experienced annual growth rates of between 30 and 40 per cent in the 1990s (Datamonitor 1998). In Europe, the UK has experienced the highest rate of growth, although other countries are now catching up. The growth in the number of telecentres is often associated with the national and international restructuring of companies whereby interaction with the customer is being shifted from face-to-face contact in high street branches to telephone operations which can be located anywhere in the country and even anywhere in the world.

Telecentre activity in Europe commenced with the selling of telephone insurance and banking in the UK and expanded to incorporate general information and inquiry calls and after sales service. The broadening role of telecentres has meant this form of working has been introduced in the UK in a diverse range of sectors including retail, leisure and tourism, transport, the utilities (gas, electricity and water) and in government offices and agencies. According to recent estimates by the research organisation Datamonitor (1998), there are currently 9,700 telecentres in Europe. This number is forecast to rise to 18,500 – employing approximately 1.3 per cent of the working population of Europe – by 2002. In the UK it is estimated that, in 1998, 250,000 or about 1.5 per cent of the working population were employed in telecentres and this is forecast to rise to 2 per cent by 2000. Approximately 45 per cent of all European telecentre agent seats are currently located in the UK. Particular regions have emerged as preferred locations, supported by central and regional government incentive packages. In the UK, the west of Scotland and Leeds have experienced particularly strong telecentre growth. There is, however, a perceived European north-south divide in the development of a teleculture, with southern European countries like Spain, France and Italy being slower at adopting telephone business than their northern European counterparts (Datamonitor 1998). Financial services industries have been most strongly associated with the development of telecentres.

A number of reports have identified the factors which are driving the development of telecentres (Income Data Services 1998; Datamonitor 1998). The most often mentioned is the perceived demand from customers to have access to services outside normal working hours. This is particularly significant because the most profitable market, with the greatest disposable earnings, is dual income families who have little time to access services within normal working hours. Cost is another major factor. The average cost of a banking transaction carried out through a telecentre is 50 per cent of that conducted face-to-face at a branch. The cost savings are obtained in three ways. First, through the use of technology which increases the efficiency of operation and enables a higher level of management control and supervision of the workforce. Second, through the savings achieved by the economies of scale and, finally, via savings in labour and overhead costs associated with locating telecentres in geographical areas where labour and space are relatively cheap.

The Technology

The efficiency of a telecentre is crucially dependent on the technology used. The most important elements are the software packages which allow a high level of automation of functions, efficient access to large databases of customer information on the part of agents and the addition of new information gathered from each customer – this is referred to as 'telecentre interaction'. The software packages also generate a high level of management information on the performance of individual telecentre agents and on the telecentre as a whole as well as enabling the setting of work performance targets by managers and supervisors.

The technology at the origin of telecentres – *automatic call distribution* (ACD)- was developed in the 1970s. ACD involved the queuing and routing of calls to agents. In subsequent versions of the technology, the agent was able to access a database record of the customer on the computer screen to obtain information and to make an entry of any transaction undertaken. This form of telecentre operation is called 'first-party call control' and is depicted diagramatically in Figure 1.

Interactive voice response units (IVRUs) allow callers to interact directly with a host computer. The most common voice response units achieve this by asking customers to press keys of touch-tone telephones. Some IVRUs, however, have voice recognition capabilities which allow the computer to recognise simple spoken commands. IVRUs can now undertake a variety of customer support functions twenty-four hours a day without the intervention of a human agent.

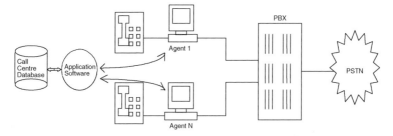

Figure 9.1 Automatic call distribution (ACD)

IVRUs often provide the first stage of customer interaction, protecting telecentre agents from having to respond to queries which they are unable to answer and which will therefore require re-routing to other agents or from having to record or give information which is sufficiently standardised to be processed automatically by the IVRU. The most efficient telecentres aim to handle eighty per cent of calls exclusively through IVRUs. They also aim to achieve an average speed of response time of fifteen seconds (the current industry average is around thirty seconds).

At the heart of the modern telecentre is *computer telephony integration* (CTI) technology. This allows voice and data information to be synchronised. It is often referred to as 'middleware'. As an agent receives a call, information regarding the customer who has made the call pops-up as a window on the agent's computer screen. The pop-up window could be triggered by the telephone number from which the call has been made. It can also be triggered by the telephone number which the customer has called – as in the case of a telecentre servicing multiple companies or multiple functions for the same company each of which has a different telephone number.

The technologies which facilitate this are referred to as automatic number identification (ANI) or calling line identification (CLI) and dialled number identification service (DNIS). ANI/CLI gives the telecentre the ability to capture the call's origin and match it against a customer database to automatically bring up on screen any records associated with the caller. DNIS, on the other hand, uses the number the caller dialled to route the call to an appropriately skilled agent, as well as informing the agent of the nature of the call. Information captured through ANI and DNIS, and any information provided by the caller during the interaction with the

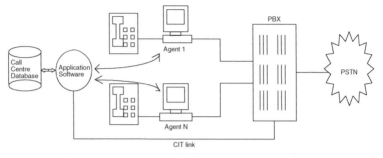

Figure 9.2 Computer-integrated telephony (CIT)

telecentre, can be matched with any pre-defined service level targets for different categories of callers, including different language requirements, or recorded as management information on agent performance. The technologies mentioned above all refer to support provided to agents dealing with incoming calls. A different set of technologies support agents involved in telesales and telemarketing campaigns.

Predictive dialling technology connects a bank of agents involved in a campaign to the database of telephone numbers to be called. As agents become available, the next number in the list is automatically called. Only if and when the call is answered will it be put through to the agent whilst simultaneously the informa-tion about the call recipient pops up on the agent's screen. Predictive dialling technology also allows an entire database of telephone numbers to be checked in advance of the start of a campaign. Each number will be annotated as to whether it is contactable or, if it cannot be contacted, the technology indicates the reason why. Whilst using manual dialling methods agents achieve a maximum 'talk time' of between fifteen and eighteen minutes per hour, with predictive dialling technology this can increase up to forty-five to fifty minutes per hour, a three-fold increase in efficiency.

The efficiency of operation of a telecentre, from the management perspective, is highly dependent on a set of software packages. These allow managers and supervisors to gain information about the operation of the centre and the performance of individual agents and to set performance targets and intervene in real time to change the way a particular sales campaign is progressing. The software allows the data obtained from customer interaction to be analysed in order to set performance targets for agents, to monitor agent performance in real time and to compare it with the achievements of other agents. Supervisors are also able to listen to agents' conversations with customers, to talk to agents during an interaction with customers without being heard and to intervene in a transaction. In summary, telecentres provide management with the potential to:

- provide improved customer service through the rapid completion of inquiries and transactions
- improve customer access by extending hours of service irrespective of time and geographical location
- achieve economies of scale in providing customer services
- rationalise operations through the removal of high volumes of customer inquiries into a single or small number of regional centres
- facilitate the re-engineering of transactions and the work processes involved in their delivery

The key management decisions concern the configuration of the telecentre operation and the handling of 'call queuing'. The optimal position is for the maximum number of staff to be working on the minimum number of queues. Multiple sites working on separate queues is generally more costly than operating with one or two sites unless the different sites can be networked together. Equally, multiple procedures and protocols operated by different telecentres is less efficient and likely to impede the intensive utilisation of telecentre capital. The current tendency, therefore, given the existing quality of the technologies available, is to concentrate telecentres in relatively large scale workplaces.

For the contemporary enterprise, the telecentre is often a catalyst of a wider strategy of organisational innovation which encompasses, for example, changing the work culture of the enterprise, the review of the product range and the review of policies concerning labour recruitment and utilisation. The culture shifts toward a strong 'customer orientation', marketing incorporates the push toward 'cross-selling' opportunities and traditional office employment patterns are displaced by more flexible working, including shiftwork, and the introduction of more varied forms of employment contract.

TECHNOLOGY, INEQUALITY AND THE
POST-INDUSTRIAL WORKPLACE

Telecentres currently require the co-location of agents in the same building. New technologies, currently being developed but still in their early stages, enable the co-ordination of the work of more than one telecentre so that tasks can be shifted from one to another according to need. This facilitates the creation of what has become known as 'virtual telecentres'. These technologies will enable people to work from home in the same way as if they were located in a telecentre. The vision of the future of the virtual telecentre is, therefore, one where individual agents will be able to work from home with their work being controlled by managers and supervisors in the same way as they are currently controlled in the physical telecentre. This will enable ultimate flexibility in the use of labour. In principle, agents could be located individually anywhere in the world and thus facilitate savings in the costs of space and other overheads. A number of experiments along these lines are currently being undertaken, but the technology is still a long way from being mature enough to allow the practical realisation of telecentres capable of delivering the economies and the flexibility which the vision foresees.

While the virtual telecentre is for the future, for the established financial services company, telecentres in the 1990s have facilitated a re-shaping of the enterprise, particularly when this technical innovation has been linked to new management techniques like human resources management (HRM), knowledge management and business process re-engineering (BPR). HRM practices have widely diffused within Europe. HRM involves team working, the identification of the workplace mission and the development of performance measurement. Knowledge management seeks to externalise the internal knowledge and skills of employees and absorb these into the systems software of the enterprise. BPR was developed by management consultants like Hammer and Champy in the US. Its purpose is not merely to use technology to replicate traditional manual systems but to deploy them to 'obliterate' traditional patterns of working (Hammer 1990; Hammer and Champy 1995). BPR's focus is the work process. It involves the establishment of work teams whose primary purpose is to redesign work processes so as to reduce wasteful procedures and duplicated effort. BPR often cuts across traditional management structures – like departments – and generates the push toward less hierarchical

190

and flatter forms of management organisation. These management techniques have been extensively adopted in telecentres in the US and UK over recent years. They attempt to secure from employees 'control through commitment' as well as 'commitment through control' and are consistent with the introduction of flatter, less hierarchical forms of management organisation.

Work Organisation: Control, Productivity and Performance

The technology of the Telecentre provides the foundation for the creation of 'factory-like' working conditions in which the non-manual worker can be subjected to the same kinds of productivity measures that were previously only applicable to their manual counterparts in goods producing industries. Management may seek to establish 'optimum' productivity and performance by identifying a combination of productivity indicators and measurement formulae:

Table 9.1 Productivity Indicators used in Telecentres

Productivity Indicators	Measurement formulae
• Number of Calls handled • Number of Callers in Queue • Average Agent Sign-On time • Agent Occupancy Percentage • Average Inbound Talk time	• Different number of hours worked by agents • Long calls v short calls • Call volume variations • Difficult v easy call

In this work environment, occupations within telecentres tend to polarise, from the management perspective, between high and low skills. Higher skilled mainly male occupations include software designers, developers and IT specialists as well as those who provide specialist advice to customers or who use, for example, language skills and lower skilled positions are typically those of mainly women agents who undertake the more 'routine' forms of customer inquiry and telesales. The routinisation of interchanges between customers and operators has become an important focus for trainers in the call centre 'industry'. Aptus is a company that provides 'bespoke' training packages for call centres. The company's training focuses on, for example, cutting the average length of calls by providing trainees with the skills required to signal the end of a call. Effective signalling, according to the managing director of Aptus, enabled one leading UK call centre company to dramatically improve productivity:

> One of the UK's largest companies (and a recent client of ours) has accomplished and maintained excellent results in their call centre productivity. A major achievement was cutting the length of the average call by 16 per cent. It means built-in growth – they can handle thousands more calls per agent.
>
> (Green 1998: 28–9)

Management consultants and trainers use training sessions to structure and discipline the thought processes involved in the exercise of mental labour; training filters out human discretion and replaces it with 'good' communications habits (Green 1998: 29).

Skill, however, is also a social construct (Ainley 1993). Management may designate certain functions, often carried out by women workers, as less skilled when, in practice, the agent at the interface between computer and customer is highly skilled in customer service provision though such skills may not be recognised or 'valued' or be properly rewarded by the enterprise. Equally, management may provide training for customer service workers that is designed to encourage the latter to use their initiative to elicit from the customer a positive or 'warm' response, a sense that the operator cares about the customer's concerns. This 'building rapport' is positively encouraged by supervisors who monitor the calls (Taylor 1998) providing, of course it produces sales for the enterprise (Farago 1998). Call centre operators are encouraged to deploy their own initiative or 'positive discretion' within a framework of a highly controlled and monitored work environment. In this sense, performance measurement enters into the social interaction between operator and customer and, arguably, constitutes a form of exploitation of emotional labour – through either the routinisation or the manipulation of emotions – that is far more insidious or invasive for the employee than the shopfloor practices associated with Taylorism and scientific management.

Geographical Location and Labour Relations

The geographical location of telecentres within the UK has typically been chosen by companies in order to maximise the potential for recruiting an 'appropriate' form of local female labour as Fincham et al (1994) recorded when interviewing management about the reasons for the Bank of Scotland establishing its VISA centre at Dunfermline:

the main reason for choosing Dunfermline was demographic. Census and population returns for the area
indicated a large supply of 'married ladies who really are
excellent workers'. The VISA centre could be staffed by
this high quality but non-career female labour force. Much
of the work available would be on a part-time basis, which
could be arranged to suit the women's domestic arrangements. There was also a strong belief amongst managers
that this expedient would solve many of the potential
health problems of working with terminals. As the operations manager put it, working on a terminal for eight
hours was really asking rather a lot of most people; part-
time work was 'more humane really'.

(Fincham et al 1994: 87)

Similar concerns occupied the Co-operative Bank when it established its customer services call centre at Skelmersdale in the early
1990s. There was a large supply of young, married female labour
living within the environs of the new town (Interview, Bank, Insurance and Finance Union (BIFU) Seconded Representative 1996). In
other financial services companies, including the Guardian Royal
Exchange (GRE) the geographical location of Guardian Direct,
established in 1994, was influenced by the character of the local
labour market. Union representatives within the company indicated that approximately 70 per cent of the total workforce within
Guardian Direct were women and GRE's call centres were considered to be 'no-go areas' for trade unionism (Interviews, GRE BIFU
Seconded Representative 1997; GRE BIFU Divisional Council
Chairperson 1997).

The experience within the UK appears to be replicated in the
European Union states according to trade union sources (PTTI
1998; FIET 1996; BIFU 1998). Typically, the following features
prevail. First, telecentres have been set-up as non-union environments either by the new entrants establishing themselves in
industries like financial services or by enterprises who deliberately
establish their telecentre operations outside of existing union
recognition and collective bargaining agreements or contract out
work to non-unionised firms. Second, a significant proportion of
telecentre staff may be on insecure employment contracts – agency,
part-time, casual or temporary – and staff turnover may be relatively high – averaging around 30 per cent per annum in UK
telecentres and slightly lower in other EU countries. Third, the

work process is typically competitive and the conditions for establishing a collective identity may be constantly undermined by the prevailing work culture and, finally, management control over operating costs, working conditions and employment practices is widely regarded as essential to the success of the workplace as a profit centre – there is, therefore, a tendency amongst management to resist attempts at unionisation.

CONCLUSION

Whilst telecentre technologies are illustrative of those typically associated with the emergence of an information society, the employment practices and working conditions are, in fact, more akin to those found on the assembly lines of the industrial factory. In short, the telecentre provides little evidence to support the optimistic scenario that the new forms of work organisation in the financial services sector founded on the extensive use of ICTs facilitate the emergence of new kinds of institutions and enterprises and new patterns of employment that achieve a decisive break with the often alienating and repetitive forms of work that were associated with the industrial 'past'.

Three features of the transformation of work thesis were identified as key themes for this chapter – the replacement of monotonous and repetitive tasks associated with assembly lines and mass production technologies by information and knowledge-based occupations that require workers to exercise discretion and responsibility; the upskilling of the workforce arising from the growth in these occupations and the breakdown of gendered divisions of labour that structure the inequalities between men and women's work.

The telecentre provides a useful test of the post-industrial thesis concerning these themes. Whilst many authors associated with this outlook argued that mass production and assembly lines were rapidly disappearing from the advanced industrial nations, they failed to recognise that many of the features of this form of work were being reproduced in the white collar factories springing up in the service sector. The telecentre, far from removing boring and monotonous jobs, has been the location in which the technical division of labour has been shaped by training schemes and software packages that sharply distinguish between high and low skilled work, with the latter often being subject to a process of routinisation embedded in the methods designed for scheduling and routing calls. As telecentres have facilitated the entrance of non-financial institutions into the financial services sector, so the increasingly competitive market conditions have pressed management into adopting measures of productivity and performance which, arguably, are more comprehensive and invasive for workers than those traditionally utilised by their counterparts in manufacturing industries. Certainly, in relation to the monitoring of performance and productivity, the embedding of monitoring methods into the software and the organisation of work has given rise to a form of management control that contains more insidious and secretive elements than those that typically prevail in many areas of manufacturing industry.

Equally, the evidence of 'up-skilling' arising from the growth of telecentres in the service sector is, at best, mixed. Undoubtedly, those who design and develop the software and manage the complex systems are skilled professional and technical staff. Nonetheless, these constitute a minority of employees. The majority of workers, particularly women workers, typically experience their work as low valued and low skilled with opportunities for staff development being confined mainly to the rotation of tasks within a narrow range of customer-oriented competencies. The consequence of this form of working, including the routinisation of what might be called emotional labour, is often low morale, high pressure and, as a result, high levels of labour turnover (Taylor 1998).

Finally, the 'white collar factory' has provided increased employment opportunities for women workers. Greenfield sites have been consciously located in urban areas where a large proportion of those available for employment are younger women workers, for whom part-time employment enables them to combine their domestic and work responsibilities (BIFU 1988; Fincham et al 1994; Poynter 2000). This rise in employment opportunities for women workers within the telecentre is part of a wider phenomenon of growth in women's employment in the UK service sector as a whole. In the 1980s and 1990s this pattern of employment growth has been analysed as a process of 'feminisation' of the workforce (Jenson et al 1988). Improved access to employment opportunities for women workers should not, however, be considered as commensurate with the achievement of greater equality between men and women at work. Financial services has for many years contained a numerical gender balance in favour of women although the majority were typically employed in lower grades, with poorer pay and few career opportunities (O'Reilly 1994). The new forms of work organisation associated with the restructuring of financial services provided an opportunity to address the traditional inequalities within the gendered division of labour. So far the opportunity has been missed. The telecentre represents a new form of work organisation in which the traditional inequalities (in recognised and valued skills, pay and benefits and working conditions) between the sexes have been largely reproduced. Some benefits, like flexible shift arrangements and childcare provision, have enabled women workers to combine domestic and work responsibilities but this has served the interests of management rather than of female labour. Short shifts at the telephonic interface with customers provide for more efficient and productive forms of working in a highly monitored and pressurised work setting.

Telecentres have emerged as a significant new form of work organisation in the service sector. They have also provided a new form of interface with customers in basic production industries – electricity, gas and water. Across several industrial sectors, the customer-oriented ethos that symbolises the work culture of the information age has created a new environment for experimentation in generating and extending new product markets. Whilst old patterns of gender inequality have been largely reproduced, telecentres have contributed toward the creation of a new work culture that, arguably, constitutes a distinctive break with traditional patterns of employment relations in large scale workplaces. In the post war period, large workplaces constituted the bedrock of blue collar trade unionism in the advanced industrial nations and, paradoxically, the small high street branch provided the focal point for the growth of white collar trade unionism amongst bank employees. The contemporary telecentre is often non-unionised and employment relations are shaped by highly competitive forms of team-working and an aggressive, competitive management style. In this new work culture, the inequalities that shaped the social and technical divisions of labour in industries like the financial services in the 1960s and 1970s have, in the 1990s, been refined and re-worked rather than modified or removed.

10

A DYNAMIC PERSPECTIVE ON TECHNOLOGY, ECONOMIC INEQUALITY AND DEVELOPMENT

Peter Senker

Technology is now enormously powerful. People travel to the moon and rockets are sent to the planets; it is possible to travel right around the world by jet airliner for less than £1,000. For a similar sum, a very powerful computer can be bought and connected to the Internet, giving access to a vast store of knowledge and information.

This chapter attempts to provide some tentative answers to a question which has worried many people for a long time: why do many millions of poor people lack the means of satisfying their most basic needs, such as nourishing food and clean water, in an era when many people have access to such powerful technological capabilities?

One of the most fundamental reasons for the persistence of large scale poverty is that the distribution of wealth and income in the world is very unequal, to the extent that there are hundreds of millions of people living in poverty and a tiny number of extremely rich people. Some indications of the extent of economic inequality follow. There are those who believe that the present economic system based on free markets works for everyone (for example, see OECD 1997). They admit that many benefits flow initially to the rich, but argue that these benefits then 'trickle down' to the poor.

There are, however, reasons to believe that this is not so. Science and technology play key roles in economic development. Forces which influence the directions in which science and technology are exploited are discussed, to try to explain why most of their benefits continue to flow to relatively affluent people. Nevertheless in the last hundred years or so, many millions have been lifted out of poverty. Some brief examples are then given of the contributions which information and communication technologies (ICTs) have made to economic growth. But other clusters of technology, such as those applied to agriculture and the development of pharmaceuticals, are significant in terms of economic growth and the distribution of its benefits and costs. Accordingly, the forces affecting the development and application of such technologies are considered, followed by a brief discussion of some significant constraints to trickle-down.

In conclusion, it is suggested that as corporations operate primarily to secure profits for their shareholders, they perceive that satisfying the needs of the hundreds of millions of relatively affluent people living in the developed world offers the most attractive markets. For this reason, they direct the research and development (R&D) they control primarily to meeting the long-term needs of those markets, and to exploitation of resources such as the biodiversity in third world countries to satisfy markets in developed countries. Such corporate behaviour represents a barrier to the development and application of technology for the relief of poverty and deprivation. Some tentative suggestions are made for tackling this enormous problem.

THE EXTENT OF WORLD POVERTY

Since 1945, the majority of the people in many industrialised nations have enjoyed substantial increases in living standards. Mass production has made available a wide range of products at prices most people in these countries can afford – from cheap clothes and food to products such as vacuum cleaners and washing machines which make household tasks less arduous. By the 1950s, most of Europe enjoyed full employment and welfare states. In the 1950s and 1960s, the end of colonialism was followed by improvements in education and health and accelerated economic development that led to dramatic declines in poverty in several developing countries.

But the advances have been very uneven (UNDP 1997: iii). In the hundred years to 1989, disparities between the income of the richest countries and the poorest widened substantially (Pritchett 1995). In the last twenty years, the disparities between the incomes of those who live in the richest countries and those in the poor developing countries where most of the world's population live have become even greater (Castells 1998: 75, 78).

This chapter is concerned with economic inequality primarily because of relationships between gross inequality in wealth and income and poverty and human deprivation in both advanced and developing countries. Poverty implies severe deprivation because poor people have access to inadequate means to pursue their well-being. Defining poverty and deprivation is not easy. Poverty can be seen as 'the failure of basic capabilities to reach certain minimally acceptable levels' (Sen 1992: 109). But the extent of the real inequality of opportunities that people face cannot be deduced from inequality of incomes alone, because what they can or cannot do or achieve depends on the various physical and social character-istics which affect their lives as well as their incomes. Low income tends to cause poverty and deprivation, but even people with rela-tively high incomes can suffer from real deprivation.

Living may be seen as consisting of a set of interrelated 'func-tionings' consisting of beings and doings. Functionings can vary from such elementary ones as being adequately nourished, being in good health, avoiding escapable morbidity and premature mortality, to complex achievements such as being happy, having self-respect, being able to appear in public without shame, and being able to take part in the life of the community.

Capability to achieve functionings depends on a wider range of factors than income. One of the most basic functionings is being able to stay alive for a reasonable length of time, and this is not solely dependent on income: Brazil has much higher income per head than China, but, on average, people live longer in China. There can even be quite remarkable differences within countries. Within India, Kerala, one of the poorer Indian states, has much higher than average life expectancy than India as a whole. Depriva-tion can affect large groups of people, even those living in the most affluent countries. Men living in Harlem in the prosperous city of New York in the United States, one of the most prosperous coun-tries in the world, have much higher incomes on average than Bangladeshi men. But they have less chance of reaching the age of 40 than Bangladeshi men because of factors such as the inadequacy of medical care and the prevalence of urban crime. Despite the fact that even the poorest groups in the United States have higher incomes than the middle classes in many poorer countries, malnu-trition persists in the United States. This is largely because hunger and malnutrition are related not only to food intake, but to the ability to make nutritious use of that intake, and this in turn is deeply affected by general health (Sen 1992).

Although the world has become much more prosperous in the last fifty years, hundreds of millions of people are still shut out from the great gains which can be secured from economic growth (UNDP 1997: 9–12). The share of world income of the poorest 20 per cent of the world's people has halved since 1960. The numbers of people who have incomes of less than one dollar a day, who lack access to clean water, and who die before they reach forty years of age each exceeds one billion. Nearly as many – more than 800 million people – are malnourished (UNDP 1999: 28). South Asia has the most people affected by poverty. Unemployment is also persistent, and low yields from subsistence agriculture and low wages in employment are major factors keeping millions of people in poverty.

There are also millions of people suffering from poverty and deprivation in advanced countries, and the proportion of the population living in poverty has increased in some Western countries. In developed countries, the adverse effects of intensified competition have tended to fall more on the poor than the rich, and on the unskilled more than on the skilled: for example, there are eighteen million unemployed in the European Union (ILO 1998: 9). Throughout the OECD area, profits have risen faster than wages since the middle of the 1970s (OECD 1994: 22–3). In most European countries, the unemployed have not benefited from general prosperity: the proceeds of economic growth have mainly been absorbed by those in employment.

Unemployment is rising in many industrial countries and traditional protections against poverty are being undermined by pressures on public welfare spending and falls in real wages. Inequality has increased markedly in some countries and effects have been worst amongst certain sections of the population – in particular amongst children, women and the aged. Eastern Europe and the Commonwealth of Independent States have suffered great increases in poverty in the last decade.

The European Commission's White Paper, *Growth, Competitiveness and Employment,* suggested that we are 'passing through a period in which there is a gap between the destruction of jobs' and 'our capacity to think up new individual or collective needs which would provide new job opportunities' (CEC 1993: 11). But the problem is not a limitation in 'our capacity to think', but in the constraints imposed on devising and implementing institutional arrangements for meeting poorer people's needs more fully. The forecasts adopted as a basis for the White Paper showed unemployment as either stable or increasing. The target of fifteen million new jobs by the year 2000 was intended to halve unemployment. To achieve it would have involved an unprecedented rate of employment creation of 2 per cent per annum (CEC 1993: 9–16). Moreover, differences in income between rich and poor regions in Europe remained substantial through the eighties. Poor regions of Europe tend to have high unemployment.

In contrast, the total wealth of the world's 358 billionaires exceeds the combined annual incomes of 45 per cent of the world's people (Elliott 1996). The world's top 500 companies employ 0.05 per cent of the world's population but control a quarter of the world's economic output. In eight sectors including cars, aerospace, electronics, steel, armaments and media, the top five corporations now control half of the global market (Vidal 1997).

THE PREVAILING IDEOLOGY

The conventional wisdom is that the development and use of new technology leads to economic development and that the benefits of economic development trickle down to benefit the whole of society. The best way to alleviate poverty is to provide the maximum freedom for individual entrepreneurs and corporations to create as much wealth as possible as quickly as possible. The poor and the poorest all benefit from wealth creation eventually because of the trickle-down of wealth and income from the rich and very rich to the poor and the very poor. Any measures which restrict entrepreneurs and corporations from pursuing competitive advantage are likely to reduce growth in wealth and income. The Organisation for Economic Co-operation and Development (OECD) is a club of the richest nations in the world. OECD policy recommendations epitomise this philosophy and influence the policies of governments and international organisations:

> An open, competitive domestic industrial base is an important means of creating jobs and enhancing public welfare. Industrial competitiveness policy helps to create conditions conducive to achieving these objectives by providing the broad framework for competitive markets.

Governments must increasingly formulate domestic policy in a global context; improve the business environment and enhance the competitiveness of markets.

(OECD 1997: 2–3)

Technological change is beneficial because declining costs of communications, transport and logistics are among the factors which can offer lower costs, better quality and more choice to consumers.

Meeting the demands of the relatively rich provides employment and thus income to the relatively poor. The creation of mass markets gives opportunity for the deployment of technology to produce high quality goods at low prices, which often benefit quite poor people. Indeed,

> benefits of intensified competition and accelerated learning are growing productivity, lower prices and a higher level of consumption ... In newly industrialised areas there may be quite dramatic increases in per capita consumption especially for the well-educated segments of the labour force.
>
> (Lundvall 1998: 5)

This prevailing ideology reached its culmination in the OECD's plans for a Multinational Agreement on Investment (MAI) (OECD 1998), which it claimed would give a new impetus to growth, employment and higher living standards. MAI would have imposed very severe restrictions on the right of any contracting state to regulate the operations of companies in its territory. For example, it would have prevented the imposition of requirements to export a given proportion of goods or services, to achieve any particular percentage of domestic content, or to transfer technology (OECD 1998: 18–20). It would have enabled multinationals to sue national governments in respect of laws which discriminate against them. It would, for example, have enabled them to challenge the UN Convention on Biological Diversity which is designed to protect developing countries' genetic resources (Rowan 1998).

There are, however, grounds for hope that the tide has turned, and that MAI has been abandoned. It was launched in 1995, at a time 'when optimism about ever-greater liberalisation was at its zenith'. A French boycott of international discussions about MAI which had been due to start again in October 1998 was reported as resulting in 'extreme pessimism' about its future amongst officials from governments involved (Elliott, Denny and Webster 1995).

TECHNOLOGY AND ECONOMIC GROWTH

Over the past several hundred years, with the aid of technology, several hundred million people have been lifted out of poverty. But why have hundreds of millions been left behind? To answer this question, it is necessary to consider the forces which drive the development of technology and its use.

Multinational corporations seek large markets because these offer the most profitable opportunities. The largest markets are offered by richer people because they have more buying power. Many large markets are offered by the relatively affluent populations who live in advanced industrial countries such as the United States, Japan and Western Europe. A high proportion of the R&D carried out in the world is directed by large multinational corporations based in advanced industrial countries such as the United States, Japan and Western Europe. Understandably, therefore, most R&D is directed by multinationals towards creating and satisfying large markets in these countries. Indeed, Whiston (1993a: 252–6) suggests that about 95 per cent of R&D is concentrated amongst Northern rich (OECD) countries, and that the vast majority of this expenditure is directed to meeting the needs of those nations. The share of developing countries in global R&D actually fell between the mid-1980s and the mid-1990s – from 6 per cent to 4 per cent (UNDP 1999: 67).

Even within Europe, R&D is very unevenly distributed: there is little or no R&D in most poor regions. Without well-developed R&D capabilities, backward regions will find it increasingly difficult to gain from advanced technology developed elsewhere. An adequate infrastructure including high quality labour and higher education institutions are prerequisites for undertaking R&D, and these also are generally lacking in poorer regions (Fagerberg, Verspagen and Caniels 1997). Corporations are directed by individuals or small groups of people. Accordingly, they vary considerably in terms of the determination, intelligence and, sometimes, ruthlessness, with which they pursue their goals (Senker 1989). However, the principal aims of all multinational corporations include making profits for their shareholders.

Having developed products and production processes to stimulate and meet the needs of the largest markets in developed countries, multinational companies then try to create and satisfy markets for those products and processes in developing countries. Their marketing and public relations include attempts to persuade governments and international organisations to create the best conditions in which those products and processes can be sold. Multinational corporations also try to persuade international organisations to lower the tariffs confronting those products and processes when they are exported to other countries, including developing countries.

INFORMATION AND COMMUNICATION TECHNOLOGIES

The development, application and use of ICTs have stimulated economic growth in numerous countries throughout the world. In advanced countries, the ICT industry has accounted for most of the recent growth in employment of highly skilled workers. Introduction of new technologies, especially computers, has been associated with increases in the skills and educational requirements of jobs, particularly in service sectors such as finance. In manufacturing, expanding use of computers and automation has continued to result in lower demand for production workers. There has been an extremely rapid rise in employment of professionals and technicians. There is a vast and growing global market for people with software skills, largely as a consequence of rapidly rising demand for software accompanied by failure to increase productivity in the production of software very quickly. These trends have resulted in persistent skills shortages (CEC 1999: 1–2).

In 1995, the developed world accounted for over three quarters of world ICT production. There are substantial markets and job opportunities emerging in the manufacture of ICT products which include telecommunication equipment, computers, defence and transportation electronics, factory automation and electronics products for use in home, office and car. Services are leading manufacturing industries in terms of their expenditure on ICT, in particular on computer services, packaged software and networks. More extensive use of ICT in service industries may result in labour-saving productivity gains and severe reductions in employment, as they have in manufacturing. There have already been severe employment reductions in sectors such as finance and insurance. There may be significant increasing employment in emerging occupations, but this tends to be hard to identify as such employment may be diffuse and unstable.

It seems likely that ICT-based innovations will require workers to have broader and higher levels of skill than in the past across a wide range of service industries in developed countries, and increasingly formal service quality standards are being articulated. This may lead to an improvement in the quality of work, as employers invest more in training in order to meet rising quality demands. However, such trends raise questions about the accessibility of such work to less qualified people. If trends in manufacturing are repeated in service industries there may be a steady erosion of demand for lower skilled workers as quality thresholds rise. Those who remain in employment need more knowledge and higher skills (Ducatel 1997).

To consider the implications of ICTs for development, it is necessary to take globalisation into account because there is an intimate and complex relationship between globalisation and the diffusion of ICTs. From an economic perspective, globalisation encompasses trade liberalisation, the removal of non-tariff barriers and the levelling of tariff rates, and involves increasing freedom of capital to move across national boundaries. Direct investment flows are generated increasingly by firms shifting production across national boundaries to locations which are most cost-effective and profitable.

In essence, economic globalisation involves the significant lowering of some important barriers which tend to prevent activities being moved around the globe. Prominent amongst these barriers are the costs of transport and communication, both of which have been falling rapidly. ICTs have played major roles in the globalisation of financial markets: they have been used to reduce the costs of communication and to increase its speed. The communication costs involved in financial markets are now so low that financial transactions can, in principle, be carried out anywhere in the world which has a modern telecommunication infrastructure. Low transport costs, low tariffs and low communication costs also remove constraints on the location of functions such as production. In an era of low costs of communication and movement of goods, competition between various locations is intensified. Intensification of international competition has been stimulated by rapid growth in world trade and international investment flows and this stimulates further diffusion of ICTs by putting pressure on corporations to cut their communication costs still further (ILO 1998: 12, 33).

Low transport and communication costs make it economic to relocate some ICT production processes to developing countries. As a consequence, demand for skills has been growing rapidly in high technology electronics production in east Asia, where the production and use of ICTs has been one of the most important means of achieving competitiveness and growth (ILO 1998: 33–41).

Software markets seem to offer particularly attractive prospects for developing countries, as the world market for software is large and growing rapidly. Several developing countries, including Chile, India, Singapore and Taiwan, have entered low-value segments of the international software export market with the expectation that cheap labour would help them to secure competitive advantage (Millar 1998). Claims processing, electronic publishing, secretarial work, airline ticketing and customer support are examples of applications being undertaken by developing countries for companies in advanced industrial countries. Taking advantage of excellent telecommunication and low wages, the eastern Caribbean carries out computer work such as data entry for many US companies. India's output of ICT products, especially software, has increased dramatically in the last decade (UNDP 1999: 61).

Production of software requires abundant resources of sophisticated skills, which India possesses as a consequence of its heavy investment in education. An additional advantage has resulted from the use of English as the language of instruction in higher education. Early success in exporting software was facilitated by economic reform which removed controls which had previously stifled enterprise, and by various measures taken by the Indian government including the provision of improved communication facilities, tax exemptions for profits from software exports, reduction of import duties and the creation of software parks. Growth of the industry was fuelled by substantial expansion in IT training financed by the Indian government, by large companies and by international organisations, which built on an infrastructure of ample supplies of an educated scientific labour force (ILO 1998: 128–9).

Although developing countries only account for a quarter of world ICT production, they have been increasing their share, especially in consumer electronics where they are responsible for nearly half of world production. Local production of both hardware and software has been made possible through the availability of a few highly educated and trained engineers supported by small skilled workforces.

TECHNOLOGIES OTHER THAN ICTS

ICTs have played major roles in the virtual eradication of poverty in the tiger economies of Singapore, Hong Kong, Taiwan and South Korea. But ICTs are not the most important technologies for developing countries. 'Information is only one of many needs. E-mail is no substitute for vaccines and satellites cannot provide clean water' (UNDP 1999: 59).

Accordingly, to try to arrive at a balanced view of the implications of technology for inequality and poverty in the world, it is necessary to take technologies other than ICTs into account, in particular agriculture which is so vital to the economies of developing countries.

Since the mid-twentieth century, a group of agricultural technologies has been developed by scientists in international research centres, adapted in national research institutions, adopted by extension agencies and agro-chemical and seed companies, and marketed to farmers. These technologies include uniform high-yield variety crops, mechanical and energy inputs and synthetic chemical pesticides – the principal means of controlling pests, especially on commercial crops. Agricultural genetic engineering is now part of this package, encompassing international legislation and trade restrictions designed to tighten corporate control over food production. Predominant agricultural development patterns and technologies have resulted in ill-effects from use of agricultural chemicals, water depletion and erosion of soil and genetic resources. These impacts raise costs to agricultural producers and undermine their profits. Despite yield increases, millions of people still go hungry (Corner House 1998).

These technologies have been developed and marketed successfully world-wide by large corporations. They have lobbied governments in favour of chemical-intensive approaches. In many countries, this chemical dependency has been encouraged by government incentives such as tax subsidies and by agricultural credit policies that require farmers to use prescribed chemicals.

Although some pesticides can help raise productivity, their continued use has had several severe adverse ecological and socio-economic effects. Farmers' costly inputs of chemicals become ineffectual and self-defeating as a consequence of pest-resistance. Many pesticides harm human health. The technologies do not meet farmers' needs and local conditions in the risk-prone diverse environments where most of the world's rural people live (Thrupp 1996: 1–7).

In countries such as the Philippines, commercial export agriculture was encouraged at the expense of subsistence food crops. Between 1960 and 1976, the acreage devoted to subsistence agriculture fell while that devoted to export crops rose (Mitter 1996). This trend has been intensified with the progressive removal of import restrictions which in the past protected domestic food producers from competition. The average household incomes of maize farmers could be reduced by as much as 30 per cent over the next six years as a consequence of cheap maize imports from the US driving down prices. This is leading to migration to commercial estates where some of the displaced may find employment as casual labourers producing fruit and vegetables for export to industrialised countries. The United States' ability to compete with maize farmers in the Philippines results more from the heavy subsidies received from the federal government than from any comparative advantage in the production of maize. Moreover, US production of maize is heavily dependent on the use of chemicals, and free trade policy has the result of providing them with substantial markets for their products (Watkins 1997).

Over the last thirty years, commercially-bred hybrid seeds have been bought by farmers from seed merchants increasingly. In northern parts of the world, almost all farmers use them. In southern countries, although non-hybrid crops are commonly used by smallholders for growing vegetables and staple foods, hybrid seeds have become the norm for many grain crops. Hybrids do not breed true in the second generation; they are either sterile or their seed is not uniformly like the parent seed and thus there is a reduction in overall performance when hybrid seed is saved and replanted. In northern countries, many farmers no longer use farm-saved seeds – partly because of lower yields but also because of the insistence of food processors and retailers on crop uniformity (Corner House 1998).

Biotechnology is likely to increase rapidly in significance in the early years of the twenty-first century. It is unlikely that poorer countries will benefit disproportionately in terms of employment: indeed, such trends as it is possible to discern indicate that advanced countries may well benefit at their expense. R&D and market potentials are concentrated in highly industrialised countries. Research tends to be concentrated in areas where it is thought likely to open up big markets in developed countries – for example to produce slow-ripening tomatoes – rather than in those which would benefit developing countries such as anti-malarial vaccines or drought-resistant crops for marginal lands.

Genetic engineering in agriculture is motivated by the aim of securing profits from rich markets in the developed world rather than by any drive to feed the hungry. Research has been directed at meeting the commercial needs of food processors rather than the nutritional needs of poorer people. For example, Monsanto's high-starch potato has been developed to make commercially-grown potatoes more suitable for the deep-fry vats of northern fast food outlets, not to be a better or cheaper food. Few of the foods produced so far or being researched and developed are foods which the hungry can afford. Moreover, the high costs of genetically-engineered crops are likely to squeeze many small farmers out of business, with the result that fewer people will be able to grow or pay for the food they need (Corner House 1998).

Genetic engineering is being used to increase poor peoples' dependence on the corporate sector for seeds, agricultural inputs and produce, reinforcing farmers' dependence on chemical herbicides and fertilizers. Like the green revolution of the 1960s and 1970s, it is liable to set in train the further evolution of plants and insects resistant to the chemicals, resulting in unprecedented pest outbreaks and weed problems. At the same time, it is likely to reduce crop biodiversity, to trigger crop failures and cause ecological degradation, thereby exacerbating the problem of food security for the poor.

A further threat posed by genetically-engineered crops to the livelihoods of small farmers arises from attempts by the industry to deny farmers the possibility of saving seeds from previous harvests, forcing them to buy their seeds annually from seed companies. Some major companies are trying to prohibit farmers from saving seed for their own use. When farmers buy seed engineered to be tolerant to the company's proprietary herbicide, Roundup, they have to sign a contract stating that they will not save any transgenic seed for the next year's planting (Lappé 1985).

There have recently been widespread protests against such policies, and they may have some effect. For example, Monsanto has bowed to pressure to renounce the 'terminator' plant technology that had led to accusations that the company was trying to dominate world food supplies by forcing farmers to buy fresh seed from it each year. Monsanto made a public commitment not to commercialise sterile seed technologies such as the one dubbed 'terminator' (Brown 1999).

Like companies operating in agricultural markets, pharmaceuticals companies are also mainly interested in large, profitable markets, and these are most readily secured by developing and marketing treatments for the illnesses prevalent in the developed world. While 18 per cent of the global disease burden is accounted for by pneumonia, diarrhœal diseases and tuberculosis, mainly in developing countries, only 0.2 per cent of the world's health-related R&D is devoted to developing treatments for these diseases (UNDP 1999: 68). Finch suggests that it is unsurprising that drug firms concentrate on the developed world's needs, such as cardio-vascular treatments, antidepressants, cholesterol-lowering drugs and ulcer-related treatments. 'Sadly, this is a commercial business,' said the UK chief executive of an international drugs company,

> We *do* concentrate on Western diseases. That is what drives us. If you want to be a major player, you have to concentrate on the big areas. There would be a lot more research into AIDS if it were as a big a problem in the western world as elsewhere.
>
> (Finch 1998)

Drug companies have developed expensive HIV treatments for rich western markets which extend the life-spans of many AIDS patients. Sufferers in developing countries cannot afford to use these medicines (Senker 1999).

The extent to which drug companies normally neglect developing countries is illustrated by an exception which proved the rule which is considered in Finch's article – a case where a drugs company is proposing to contribute generously to the cure of elephantiasis, a disease which affects developing countries. Elephantiasis is a crippling and disfiguring tropical disease whose grotesque effects result in sufferers becoming social outcasts. It affects 120 million people, and more than one billion are at risk of contracting it. SmithKlineBeecham (SKB) announced it was to

donate one billion pounds over twenty years to a project designed
to eradicate it by 2020 (Finch 1998).

> The three drugs used to treat elephantiasis are out of
> patent and individually cost less than 10p [pence] each.
> Although SKB might lose some £50 million a year over 20
> years, this is seen as a small price to pay for the humani-
> tarian kudos it will garner.
>
> (Mihill 1998)

Several multinational companies are at present exploring and
seeking to exploit the biodiversity of the developing world. In
particular, they are seeking to exploit the potential of the active
ingredients of plants used in traditional herbal medicine. Through
patent protection, they seek to appropriate traditional remedies for
exploitation in developed countries which offer the most profit
potential, and try to prevent people in the developing world from
using their traditional remedies. The neem tree, which yields
natural pesticides and medicines and which has been used by
Indian villagers for over two thousand years, is a prime example.
Chewing neem tree shoots protects teeth from bacteria. Indian
cottage industries have been selling neem products for forty years,
and Calcutta Chemicals has been selling neem toothpaste for
decades. Since 1985, however, several patents have been taken out
by US and Japanese companies for exclusive rights to neem tree
products. Such patents are supported by a multilateral agreement
on intellectual property – Trade-Related Aspects of Intellectual
Property Rights (TRIPS) – which came into effect under the World
Trade Organisation (WTO) which was established in 1994. The
Neem Campaign was initiated in 1993 in India to mobilise world-
wide support to protect the neem tree from piracy by western and
Japanese companies utilising property rights regimes established
under WTO and TRIPS (UNDP 1999: 67).

Major corporations seeking competitive advantage are also
likely to introduce a wide range of new materials which have
performance advantages over traditional materials. Those likely to
have the most impact include strong engineering plastics, adhe-
sives, composite materials and advanced high performance
technical ceramics. The leading countries in the exploitation of
new materials are likely to be Japan and the United States,
followed by Germany. Most estimates and forecasts show Japanese
production accounting for about half of a rapidly growing world

market for advanced ceramics in the next decade. There is no evidence so far that developing countries will benefit substantially (Senker 1995).

CONSTRAINTS ON TRICKLE-DOWN

In advanced countries, high technology ICT products and services are initially bought mainly by people with high incomes, and then diffuse rapidly to most of the rest of society as economies of scale in their production rapidly make them cheaper. But rapid diffusion depends on a relatively equal pattern of income distribution. Latin American countries have average incomes about a seventh of those in advanced countries. Few people, therefore, can afford the rapid succession of high technology goods which are continually introduced into advanced countries' markets and diffuse rapidly within them. As a consequence, the introduction of high technology goods and services has had only a very slight impact on the well-being of the general population in Latin America (Dagnino and Thomas 1998).

A further significant barrier to the development of ICT industries in developing countries relates to the difficulties of transferring knowledge between software producers in developing countries and their clients in the developed countries to whom they export. Research has shown that learning and innovation results from interactions between software producers and users. Innovation provides a foundation on which international competitiveness and new opportunities for trade can be built. Such conditions rarely exist in developing countries such as India which generally lack thriving technologically sophisticated domestic markets for software. Constraints on learning from users in developing countries result in domestic producers failing to secure a strong foundation for competing in the higher value-added segments of the international software market.

Knowledge inputs to software development are context-specific, and the learning process through which software producers must progress takes place most effectively if the producers are physically located near the users. It has been suggested that producers can only learn from users if they all operate in the same environment with common characteristics which facilitate effective communication, such as language, legal and educational systems, work organisation, and even religion. Such factors constrain developing countries' share of total world software production and trade (Millar 1998).

As shown above, the low communication costs afforded by advanced telecommunication systems do create some opportunities for countries which have cheap resources of highly skilled labour to compete with more expensive skilled labour elsewhere. ICTs have played, and will probably continue to play, significant roles in stimulating economic growth in many countries. But constraints on producers in developing countries learning from users result in domestic producers failing to secure a strong foundation for competing in the higher value-added segments of the international software market. Extreme doubts have been expressed about the feasibility of overcoming such constraints. Advanced countries still dominate production and use of higher value-added ICTs, and examples of economic success in developing countries are both exceptional and very small in scale in comparison with the extent of world poverty.

While markets for goods and services are becoming increasingly globalised – especially in relation to ICTs – international trade, investment and financial flows are concentrated in Europe, Japan and North America, and this dominance seems likely to continue. Real commodity prices in the 1990s were much lower than in the 1980s. The terms of trade for the least developed countries have deteriorated substantially over the past twenty-five years. Average tariffs on industrial country imports from the least developed countries are much higher than the global average. Developing countries lose about $60 billion a year from agricultural subsidies and barriers to textile imports in industrial countries. The Uruguay Round (of tariff reductions) left most of the protection for industry and agriculture in industrial countries intact. Tariffs are much higher for the goods with the greatest potential for the poorest countries such as agricultural commodities, textiles and leather. The United States and the European Union have applied anti-dumping measures against a wide range of developing country exports – everything from steel to colour television and toys. There is little enthusiasm for removing the bias in the rules of international trade in favour of industrialised countries in relation to barriers to international trade. Two-thirds of foreign direct investment in developing countries has gone to only eight countries, and half of developing countries have received hardly any foreign direct investment at all (UNDP 1997: 9).

With the exception of a small minority of newly industrialising countries, the Third World remains marginal in respect of both investment and trade: capital mobility is not producing a massive shift of investment from advanced to developing countries, and labour mobility between countries and regions is very low (Hirst and Thompson 1996: 2–6, Castells 1996: 95, Waters 1995: 93). Research and development relevant to meeting the basic needs of the majority of the world's population in areas such as food agriculture and shelter is grossly neglected (Whiston 1993).

CONCLUSIONS

Technological change stimulated by competitive markets has been instrumental in achieving substantial increases in the living standards of the majority of people in developed countries. But hundreds of millions of people are shut out from the great gains which can be achieved from economic growth and technological change. In general, technological change is being guided in directions which represent a continuing process of favouring already affluent people and regions. A high proportion of the world's R&D is carried out by large multinational companies in pursuit of profits. Understandably, major corporations place the vast majority of their R&D investments in projects which they perceive as likely to yield them the greatest long-term profits – in applications where there are large potential markets of relatively rich consumers with high disposable incomes who can afford to buy the products which are developed.

The trickle-down theory assumes that unregulated markets are always beneficial because firms compete to meet customers' needs, and competition results in the production of high quality low-cost products. Consumers everywhere benefit from buying low-cost products wherever they are made. But this theory does not allow for the real possibility that some products and processes developed primarily for the benefit of affluent people threaten the livelihoods of poor people in developing countries.

In agriculture, far from corporations competing to meet customers' needs, people in many developing countries have fought corporations supported by governments to introduce sustainable agricultural practices – in particular integrated pest management (IPM) which can be beneficial to farmers' profitability and the welfare of the population in general (Watkins 1997). Similarly, the

Neem Campaign tries to protect indigenous knowledge systems and resources of the Third World multinational corporations who wish to exploit these resources for the benefit of their largest markets in the developed world (Shiva 1997).

R&D directed at the improvement of the standard of living of subsistence farmers has very low priority for corporations, as potential markets are perceived as too small and heterogeneous to justify significant expenditures. Genetic engineering is unlikely to be developed primarily to help stave off world starvation, because poor people cannot offer profitable markets. On the contrary, application of genetic engineering is liable to threaten crop yields, to force farmers to pay for their rights to fertile seed, to reduce foreign demand for some Third World produce and to contribute to environmental degradation (Corner House 1998).

Multinational corporations and protesters against their policies are both rational, but corporations and protesters are operating under different logics. Disputes mainly arise because the logic under which multinational corporations operate – the search for profits – dictates that they seek to develop and exploit the largest markets, and direct their R&D towards those objectives. Once multinational corporations have developed products and processes which have large markets in the developed world, they seek to secure further profits by exploiting their products and processes in the developing world. Similarly, when corporations become aware of assets in developing countries, their primary goal is to exploit them in the developed world, principally because wealthier countries offer larger markets.

The ideology sustaining the views and policies of organisations such as OECD and WTO is that unbridled international competition will lead to trickle-down of wealth and income from rich to poor. Trickle-down does occur to a considerable extent and, indeed, has been responsible over the years for bringing hundreds of millions of people out of poverty. But corporations direct the R&D they control primarily to meeting the long term needs of markets in developed countries, and exploitation of resources such as the biodiversity in third world countries to satisfy larger markets in developed countries.

Technology has not succeeded in eliminating poverty mainly because the alleviation of poverty is not a major goal of those who direct multinational corporations which play such a large role in directing the world's technological efforts. Protests may sometimes succeed in stopping the exploitation of technologies which people in both developed and developing countries regard as undesirable. International regulation could possibly be designed to play a far greater role in controlling the inappropriate exploitation of technology. Technologies are rarely good or bad in themselves. There are opportunities for developing and shaping them in various ways. For example, in relation to genetically modified crops, Sir Robert May, the British government's chief scientist, was reported as saying,

> It seems unclear, at this point, whether GM crops have the potential to be a further notch up in (agricultural) intensification and as such, not good. But equally, they have the potential to enable us to redesign crops so that we work with nature and shape the crops to the environment rather than shape the environment to the crops in ways which are unsustainable ... I take a rather different view of this from Greenpeace, who see it as a prime campaign issue and necessarily bad.
>
> (May, quoted in Douglas 1999)

Development and exploitation of new technology is extremely expensive. In the current world market regime, no way has yet been found of directing technology towards the alleviation of poverty. This has the consequence of depriving millions of very poor people of possibilities for substantial improvement of their lives through the application of technology.

It is unreasonable to look to the workings of unregulated free markets to play the main role in alleviating world poverty and deprivation. Major multinational corporations, the principal players in the world's markets, do not pursue the objective of alleviating world poverty, primarily because they are essentially market-creating and market-satisfying organisations. They neglect the poor not because corporations are inherently evil, but because the poor do not offer attractive markets.

Technological development could conceivably be used to alleviate poverty much more rapidly. But this would require much stricter and more coherent regulation of international finance, trade, agriculture and industry in the interests of the world's poor than has so far been contemplated. Even such measures might well be inadequate, as regulation is only capable of preventing technology from being used inappropriately. Means for deploying substantial technological resources positively towards the alleviation of deprivation and poverty under international control are surely worthy of consideration. This could involve major changes in the goals and operations of existing international organisations, and, quite possibly, the creation of new ones. It would also involve the abandonment of policies based on trickle-down on the basis of its demonstrated inadequacy, and their replacement by policies based on significant transfer of resources from rich to poor. The adoption of such policies on an international basis would require massive political barriers to be surmounted.

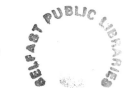

BIBLIOGRAPHY

Abramovitz, M.A. (1986) 'Catching up, forging ahead and falling behind', *Journal of Economic History* 46: 385–406.
Adam, A. and Green, E. (1998) 'Gender, agency, location and the new information society' in B.D. Loader (ed.) *Cyberspace Divide. Equality, Agency and Policy in the Information Society*, London: Routledge.
Ainley P. (1993) *Class and Skill: Changing Divisions of Knowledge and Labour*, London: Cassell.
Allen, R. (1999) 'Cyberchimeras: media self-regulation paradigms for the Internet', in R. Allen, T. Holmes and A. Phillips (eds) *Self Regulation in the Media*, 83–96 Edinburgh: Merchiston Press.
Amsden, A. (1991) 'Diffusion of development; the late industrialising model and Greater East Asia', *American Economic Review* 81,2: 282–6.
– (1992) 'A theory of government interaction in late industrialisation', in L. Putterman and D. Rueschmeyer (eds) *The State and Market in Development*, New York: Lynn Riener.
Amsden, A. and Hikino, T. (1991) 'Borrowing technology or innovating: an exploration of two paths to industrial development', *Working Paper No.3*, New York: New School for Social Research.
Anderson, C. (1975) *Video Power: Grassroots Television*, New York: Praeger.
Ang, I. (1991) *Desperately Seeking the Audience*, London: Routledge.
– (1996) *Living Room Wars: Rethinking Media Audiences for a Postmodern World*, London: Routledge.
Arnot, M. (1995) 'Bernstein's theory of educational codes and feminist theories of education: a personal view', in A. Sadovik (ed.) *Knowledge and Pedagogy: The Sociology of Basil Bernstein*, Norwood: Ablex Publishing Corp.
Association of Progressive Communications (1999) Online. Available HTTP: http://www.apc.org (20 October 1999).
Bairoch, P. (1981) 'The main trends in national economic disparities since the industrial revolution', in P. Bairoch and M. Levy-Loboyen (eds) *Disparities in Economic Development since the Industrial Revolution*, London: Macmillan.
Bank for International Settlements (BIS) (1998), *68th Annual Report*, Basle: BIS.

Banking, Insurance and Finance Union (BIFU) (1984) *Jobs for the Girls? The Impact of Automation on Women's Jobs in the Finance Industry*, London: BIFU.

– (1988) *The Monopolies and Mergers Commission Enquiry into Credit Card Services: Submission of the Banking Insurance and Finance Union*, London: BIFU.

– (1998) 'Organising Telephone Call Centres', *New Unionism Seminar Report*, London: BIFU.

Barbrook, R. (1996) 'Global algorithm 1.5: hypermedia freedom', *CTHEORY – Theory, Technology and Culture* 19,1–2. Online. Available HTTP: http://www.ctheory.com/ga1.1–hyper_freedom.html (19 October 1999).

– (1998) 'The hi-tech gift economy', *First Monday* 3,12. Online. Available HTTP: http://www.firstmonday.dk/issues/issue3_12/barbrook/index.html (19 October 1999).

Barlow, J.P. (1996) 'A declaration of the independence of cyberspace'. Online. Available HTTP: http://www.eff.org/pub/Publications/John_Perry_Barlow/barlow_0296.declaration (19 October 1999).

– (1998) 'Africa rising', *Wired,* January: 142–58.

Battersby, K. (1999) 'It's a beautiful game … of two halves and low screen options', *Evening Standard* (23 August).

Baumol, H. and Baumol, W.J. (1983) 'The mass media and the cost disease', in W.S. Hendon, D.V. Shaw and N. K. Grant (eds) *Economics of Cultural Industries*, Akron: Association for Cultural Economics.

Bell D. (1973) *The Coming of Post-Industrial Society*, New York: Basic Books.

– (1980) 'The social framework of the information society', in T. Forester (ed.) *The Microelectronics Revolution*, Oxford: Blackwell.

Benjamin, W. (1969) *Illuminations*, trans. H. Zohn, New York: Schocken Books.

Bernstein, B. (1990) *The Structuring of Pedagogic Discourse: Class, Codes and Control*, London: Collier-Macmillan.

Berry, B. J. L., Harpham, E. J and Elliott, J. F. (1994) 'Long swings in American inequality, the Kuznets conjecture revisited', mimeo, University of Texas at Dallas.

Bijker, W.E. (1995) *Of Bicycles, Bakelites and Bulbs, Toward a Theory of Sociotechnical Change*, Cambridge, MA: MIT Press.

Blaine, K. (1983) 'The September purge', *Fuse* 7, 1–2: 54–9.

Blumler J.G. and Nossiter T.J. (1991) *Broadcasting Finance in Transition*, Oxford: Oxford University Press.

Borsook, P. (1996) 'Cyberselfish', *Mother Jones*, July/August. Online. Available HTTP: http://www.motherjones.com/mother_jones/JA96/borsook.html (23 November 1999).

Boston, W. (1999) 'Kirch, BSkyB Pay-TV talks heat up', *The Wall Street Journal Europe* (4 November).

Bourdieu, P. (1984) *Distinction*, London: Routledge & Kegan Paul.

Bradley, H. (1996) *Fractured Identities: Changing Patterns of Inequality*, Cambridge: Polity.

Brecht, B. (1930) 'Radio', in A. Mattelart and S. Siegelaub (eds) (1983) *Communication and Class Struggle: Volume 2*, New York: IMMRC/ International General.

British Broadcasting Corporation (BBC) (1994) *BBC Handbook 93–4 Incorporating the Annual Report and Accounts*, London: BBC.

Brown, P. (1999) 'GM giant climbs down', *The Guardian* (5 October).

Burnaby Community TV (1992) *Women in Media*, Burnaby, B.C.: Rogers Cable TV, Transmission (September).

Burnett, R. (1991) 'Video/Film: from communication to community', in N. Thede and A. Ambrosi (eds) *Video the Changing World*, Montreal: Black Rose Books.

Calhoun, C. (ed.) (1992) *Habermas and the Public Sphere*, Cambridge, MA: MIT Press.

Canadian Radio, Television and Telecommunications Commission (CRTC) (1988) *Balance in Programming on Community Access Media*, Public Notice 1988–161, Ottawa: CRTC.

– (1989–90) *Rogers Vancouver Licence File 1989–1990*, Vancouver: CRTC.

– (1990) *Review of Community Channel Policy*, Public Notice 1990–57, Ottawa: CRTC.

Cardiff, D. and Scannell, P. (1987) 'Broadcasting and national unity', in J. Curran, Smith and P. Wingate (eds) *Impacts and Influences: Essays on Media Power in the Twentieth Century*, London: Routledge.

Carver, R. (1992) *Interview*, Programme Director, East Vancouver Neighbourhood TV, Vancouver: Rogers Cablevision (7 October).

Castells, M. (1989) *The Informational City*, Oxford: Blackwell.

– (1996) *The Rise of the Network Society*, Oxford: Blackwell.

– (1997) *The Power of Identity*, Oxford: Blackwell.

– (1998) *End of Millennium*, Oxford: Blackwell.

Central Statistical Office (CSO) (1995) *Social Trends*, London: CSO.

Cerf, V. (1999) 'The Internet is for everyone', speech given at the Computers, Freedom and Privacy conference, April. Online. Available HTTP: http://www.istf.isoc.org/archive/net4all.shtml (19 October 1999). Reprinted in *On the Internet* July/August 1999: 8–9.

Chippindale, P. and Franks, S. (1991) *Dished! The Rise and Fall of British Satellite Broadcasting*, London: Simon and Schuster.

Clark C. (1940) *The Conditions of Economic Progress*, London: MacMillan.

Cleveland-Peck, P. and Hammersley, B. (1999) 'Sky scores at both ends with replay gimmick', *The Times Interface*, (25 August).

Cockburn, C. (1983) *Brothers: Male Dominance and Technological Change*, London: Pluto.

– (1985) *Machinery of Dominance: Women, Men and Technical Knowhow*, London: Pluto.

Cole, A., Conlon, T., Jackson, S. and Welsh, D. (1994) 'Information technology and gender: problems and proposals', *Gender and Education* 6,1: 77–86.

Collins, R. (1990) *Television: Policy and Culture*, London: Unwin Hyman.

Commission of the European Communities (CEC) (1993) *White Paper: Growth, Competitiveness, Employment: The Challenges and Ways Forward into the 21st Century*, Luxembourg: Office for Official Publications of the European Communities.

– (1997a) *Protocol to the Amsterdam Treaty on June 1997, On the System of Public Broadcasting in the Member States*. Online. Available HTTP: http://www.poptel.org.uk/carole-tongue/pubs/potocol.html (15 February 1999).

– (1997b) *Green Paper on the Convergence of the Telecommunications, Media and Information Technology Sectors, and the Implications for regulation. Towards an Information Society Approach*. Online. Available HTTP: http://www.ispo.cec.be/convergencegp/97623.html (27 April 1998).

– Directorate of Culture and Audiovisual Policy (1997) *The European Film Industry under Analysis. Second Information Report 1997*. Online. Available HTTP: http://europa.eu.int/comm/dg10/avpolicy/key_doc/ cine97_e.html (27 October 1999).

– High Level Group on Audiovisual Policy (1998) *The Digital Age – European Audiovisual Policy*. Online. Available HTTP: http://europa.eu.int/comm/dg10/avpolicy/key_doc/htg_en.html (27 October 1999).

– Submission by Carole Tongue, MEP, Chair of the Cinema and Audiovisual Intergroup of the European Parliament (1998) *Audiovisual Communications and Broadcasting Regulation in the Light of Convergence*. Online. Available HTTP: http://www.poptel.org.uk/carole-tongue/pubs/converg3.html (15 February 1999).

– Directorate of Employment and Social Affairs (1999) *ESF Info Review*, Luxembourg: Office for Official Publications of the European Communities.

Consumers' Association (1998) *Which? Online Annual Internet Survey Report*, London: Consumers' Association.

Cook, P.G. and Ruggles, M.A. (1992) 'Balance and freedom of speech: challenge for Canadian broadcasting', *Canadian Journal of Communication* 17: 37–59.

Corner House (1998) *Food? Health? Hope?: Genetic Engineering and World Hunger*, Sturminster Newton: Corner House.

Cressey, P. and Scott, P. (1992) 'Employment, technology and industrial relations in the UK clearing banks: is the honeymoon over?', *New Technology, Work and Employment* 7, 2: 83–97.

Crompton R. and Jones G. (1984) *White Collar Proletariat, Deskilling and Gender in Clerical Work*, London: MacMillan.

Curran, J. (1991) 'Rethinking the media as public sphere', in R. Dahlgren and C. Sparks (eds) *Communication and Citizenship*, London: Routledge.

Curran, J. and Seaton, J. (1997) *Power without Responsibility*, 5th ed. London: Routledge.

Dagnino, R. and Thomas, H. (1998) 'Latin American science and technology policy: new scenarios and the research community', paper presented at EASST conference, Lisbon, October.

Dahlgren, P. (1995) *Television and the Public Sphere: Citizenship, Democracy and the Media*, London: Sage.

Dain, J. (1992) 'Person-friendly computing', paper presented at the Women into Computing conference, 'Teaching Computing: Contents and Methods', Staffordshire, July.

Datamonitor (1998) *Call Centre Technology in Europe*, London: Datamonitor.

Deep Dish TV (1991) *Pamphlet*, New York: Deep Dish TV.

Dempsey, L. (1993) 'Research networks and academic information services: towards an academic information infrastructure', *Journal of Information Networking*, 1,1: 1–27.

Department for Education and the Environment (DfEE) (1997a) *Report of the National Inquiry into Higher Education: Higher Education in the Learning Society (The Dearing Report)*, London: HMSO.

– (1997b) *Connecting the Learning Society: National Grid for Learning*, London: HMSO.

– (1998) *The Learning Age: A Renaissance for a New Britain*, London: HMSO.

Department of National Heritage (1992) *The Future of the BBC: A Consultation Document*, CM 2098, London: HMSO.

Depres C. and Hiltrop, J.-M. (1995) 'Human resource management in the knowledge age, current practice and perspectives on the future', *Employee Relation* 17,1: 9–23.

Dicken P. (1992) *Global Shift: The Internationalisation of Economic Activity*, 2nd ed. London: Chapman and Hall.

Dolan, E. (1984) *TV or CATV? The Struggle for Power*, Port Washington, NY: Associated Faculty Press.

Douglas, E. (1999) 'The Guardian profile Robert May: Testing, testing', *The Guardian* (30 October).

Dowmunt, T. (ed.) (1993) *Channels of Resistance: Global Television and Local Empowerment*, London: BFI in association with Channel Four.

DP Connect (1997) *Women in IT Campaign Brief*, Bromley: DP Connect.

Drucker, P. (1986) *The Frontiers of Management*, New York: Dutton.

Ducatel, K. (1997) *Unexpected Innovations: The Future of Work in Non-Technology Based Services*, Sevilla: IPTS-JRC.

Economist (1999) 'The Best-Laid Plans' (25 September).

Elliott, L. (1996) 'Holding the short straw; global equality will drive next phase of industrial revolution?', *The Guardian* (5 August).

Elliott, L., Denny, C. and Webster, P. (1998) 'Investment pact in tatters', *The Guardian* (15 October).

Ellul, J. (1964) *The Technological Society*, trans. J. Wilkinson, New York: Knopf (first published in 1954).

Enzensberger, H.M. (1976) *Raids and Reconstructions*, London: Pluto.

Ess, C. (1994) 'The political computer: hypertext, democracy and Habermas' in G. Landow (ed.) *Hyper/Text/Theory*, Baltimore, MD: Johns Hopkins University Press.

Euromedia Research Group (1992) *The Media in Western Europe: The Euromedia Handbook*, London: Sage.

Fagerberg, J., Verspagen, B. and Caniels, M. (1997) 'Technology, growth and unemployment across European regions', *Regional Studies* 31,5: 457–66.

Farago R. (1998) 'The customer is not *your* friend', *Call Centre Europe* 20: 42–6.

Ferry, J. (1996) 'Digital television: Sky's final frontier', *Business Age* April.

FIET (International Federation of Commercial, Clerical, Professional and Technical Employees) (1996) *Teleworking and Trade Union Strategy*, Geneva: FIET.

Finch, J. (1998) 'Last of the billion dollar drugs', *The Guardian* (31 January).

Fincham, R., Fleck, J., Procter, R., Scarbrough, H., Tierney, M. and Williams R. (1994) *Expertise and Innovation, Information Technology Strategies in the Financial Services Sector*, Oxford: Clarendon.

Fisher, A. (1939) 'Production: primary, secondary and tertiary', *The Economic Record* 15: 24–38.

Freeman, C. (1987) 'The case for technological determinism' in R. Finnegan, G. Salaman and K. Thompson (eds) *Information Technology: Social Issues, A Reader*, Sevenoaks: Hodder & Stoughton.

Fryer, R.H. (1997) *Learning in the Twenty-first Century: Report of the National Advisory Group for Continuing Education and Lifelong Learning*, London: HMSO.

Galbraith, J.K. (1993) *A Short History of Financial Euphoria*, Harmondsworth: Penguin.

Gallie, D. (1996) 'Skill, gender and the quality of employment', in R.Crompton, D. Gallie and K. Purcell (eds) *Changing Forms of Employment*, London: Routledge.

Game, A. and Pringle, R. (1984) *Gender at Work*, London: Pluto.

Garnham, N. (1986a) 'The media and the public sphere', in P. Golding, G. Murdock and P. Schlesinger (eds) (1986) *Communicating Politics: Mass Communications and the Political Process*, Leicester: Leicester University Press.

– (1986b) 'The media and the public sphere', *Intermedia* 14,1: 47–62.

– (1989) 'Has public service broadcasting failed?', in N. Miller and C. Norris (eds) *Life After the Broadcasting Bill*, Manchester: Manchester Monographs.

– (1990) *Capitalism and Communication*, London: Sage Publications.

Garnham, N. and Locksley, G. (1991) 'The economics of broadcasting', in J.G. Blumler and T.J. Nossiter (eds) *Broadcasting Finance in Transition*, Oxford: Oxford University Press.

Gaynor, D. (1997) Democracy in the Age of Information: A Reconception of the Public Sphere. Washington DC: Online. Available HTTP: http://www.georgetown.edu/bassr/gaynor/intro.htm (10 May 1998)

Georgia Technical University (1999) *Internet User Surveys*. Online. Available HTTP: http://www.cc.gatech.edu/gvu/user_surveys (20 October 1999).

Gershuny J. and Miles I. (1983) *The New Service Economy: The Transformation of Employment in Industrial Societies*, London: Francis Pinter.

Giddens, A. (1976) *New Rules of Sociological Method*, London: Hutchinson.

– (1984) *The Constitution of Society: Outline of a Theory of Structuration*, Cambridge: Polity.

Gillespie, G. (1975) *Public Access Cable Television in the United States and Canada*, New York: Praeger.

Goldberg, K. (1990) *The Barefoot Channel: Community Television as a Tool for Social Change*, Vancouver: New Star Books.

Golding, P. (1990) 'Political communication and citizenship: the media and democracy in an egalitarian social order', in M. Ferguson (ed.) *Public Communication: The New Imperatives*, London: Sage.

Green, J. (1998) 'Save seconds: teach them how to say goodbye', *Call Centre Europe* 20: 28–9.

Gregory, A. and O'Reilly, J. (1996) 'Checking out and cashing up' in R. Crompton, D. Gallie and K. Purcell (eds) *Changing Forms of Employment*, London: Routledge.

Grint, K. and Gill, R. (eds) (1995) *The Gender-Technology Relation*, London: Taylor & Francis.

Groombridge, B. (1972) *Television and the People: A Programme for Democratic Participation*, Harmondsworth: Penguin.

Grossman, L. (1995*) The Electronic Republic: Reshaping Democracy in the Information Age*, New York: Viking.

Guardian (1999) 'Prime minister takes first steps on road to email and the Internet' (25 October).

Habermas, J. (1974) 'The public sphere: an encyclopedia article (1964)', *New German Critique* 14: 49–55.

–(1979) *Communication and the Evolution of Society*, trans. T. McCarthy, Boston: Beacon Press (first published in German in 1976).

– (1989), *The Structural Transformation of the Public Sphere*, trans. T. Burger and F. Lawrence, Cambridge, MA: MIT Press (first published in German in 1962).

– (1990) 'Discourse Ethics: Notes on Philosophical Justification' in *Moral Consciousness and Communicative Action*, 43–115. Cambridge, MA: MIT Press.

Hacker, S. (1989) *Pleasure, Power and Technology*, London: Unwin Hyman.

– (1990) 'Mathematization of engineering: limits on women and the field', in D.E. Smith and S. M. Turner (eds) *Doing it the Hard Way: Investigations of Gender and Technology*, London: Unwin Hyman.

Hafner, K. and Lyon, M. (1996) *Where Wizards Stay Up Late: The Origins of the Internet*, New York: Simon & Schuster.

Hall, P. (1991) 'A new strategy for the South East', *The Planner*, March: 6–9.

Hamel G. and Prahalad C. (1996) 'Competing in the new economy: managing out of bounds', *Strategic Management Journal* 17: 237–42.

Hammer M. (1990) 'Re-engineering work: Don't automate, obliterate', *Harvard Business Review*, July-August: 104–12.

Hammer, M. and Champy, J. (1995) *Re-engineering the Corporation*, London: Beasley.

Handy, C. (1995) 'The Future of Work', *WH Smith Contemporary Papers* 8.

Haraway, D. (1985) 'A manifesto for cyborgs: science, technology and socialist feminism in the 1980s', *Socialist Review* 15,2: 65–108.

– (1997) *Modest_Witness @ Second_Millennium*, New York: Routledge.

Hardin, H. (1985) *Closed Circuits: The Sell-out of Canadian Television*, Toronto & Vancouver: Douglas & MacIntyre.

Hayes, D. (1999) 'Programme trade deficit soars as the UK struggles to tap potential markets overseas: learning to sell British television', *Sunday Business* (30 May).

Haywood, T. (1998) 'Global networks and the myth of equality: trickle down or trickle away?' in B.D. Loader (ed) *Cyberspace Divide. Equality, Agency and Policy in the Information Society*, London: Routledge.

Head, S. (1996) 'The New Ruthless Economy', *New York Review of Books* (29 February).

Henderson J. (1989) *The Globalisation of High Technology Production*, London: Routledge.

Henwood, F. (1993) 'Establishing gender perspectives on information technology: problems, issues and opportunities' in E. Green, J. Owen and D. Pain (eds), *Gendered by Design? Information Technology and Office Systems*, London: Taylor & Francis.

– (1996) 'WISE Choices? understanding occupational decision-making in a climate of equal opportunities for women in science and technology', *Gender and Education* 8,2: 199–214.

– (1998) 'Engineering difference: discourses on gender, sexuality and work in a college of technology', *Gender and Education* 10,1: 35–49.

Hill, C. (1997) *Attention! Production! Audience! Performing Video in its First Decade, 1968–1980*. Antioch, NY: Antioch College. Online. Available HTTP: http://www.nomadnet.org/massage1/ (1 September 2000).

Hill, S. (1999) 'Exorcising the demon', *Internet Magazine* 58 September: 42–6.

Hills, J. with Papathanassopoulos, S. (1991) *The Democracy Gap: The Politics of Information and Communication Technologies in the United States and Europe*, London: Greenwood Press.

Hirschhorn L. (1984) *Beyond Mechanisation: Work and Technology in a Post-Industrial Age*, Cambridge, MA: MIT Press.

Hirst, P. and Thompson, G. (1996) *Globalization in Question*, Cambridge: Polity.

Hobday, M. (1995) *Innovation in East Asia: The Challenge to Japan*, Aldershot: Elgar.

Hoffman, D.L. and Novak, T.P. (1998) 'Bridging the digital divide: The impact of race on computer access and Internet use', *Working Paper*, Nashville: Vanderbilt University. Online. Available HTTP: http://www2000.ogsm.vanderbilt.edu (19 October 1999).

Hoffman-Reim, W. (1993) 'The broadcasting activities of the European Community and their implications for national broadcasting systems in Europe', *Hastings International and Comparative Law Review*, 16,4: 599–617.

Hohendahl, P. (1979) 'Critical theory, public sphere and culture: Jürgen Habermas and his critics', *New German Critique* 19: 89–118.

Holderness, M. (1998) 'Who are the world's information-poor?' in B.D. Loader (ed.) *Cyberspace Divide. Equality, Agency and Policy in the Information Society*, London: Routledge.

Hollins, T. (1984) *Beyond Broadcasting: Into the Cable Age*, London: BFI Publishing.

Home Office (1982) *Report of the Inquiry into Cable Expansion and Broadcasting Policy*, CMND 8679, London: HMSO.

– (1986) *Report of the Committee on Financing the BBC*, CMND 9824, London: HMSO.

Horwitz, R. (1991) 'The First Amendment meets some new technologies: broadcasting, common carriers, and free speech in the 1990s', *Theory and Society*, 20: 21–72.

Hosking, P. (1999) 'Here is the news: ITV after 9pm has been a bit disappointing', *Evening Standard* (12 May).

Hudson, D. (1997) *Rewired: A Brief (and opinionated) Net History*, Indianapolis: Macmillan Technical Publishing.

Hughes, T. (1999) 'Technological progress has left majority in the dark', *The Times* (20 September).

Huitema, C. (1998) *IPv6: The New Internet Protocol*, 2nd ed., New Jersey: Prentice-Hall.

Iannotta, B. (1999) 'Earth, you've got mail', *New Scientist* 22 May: 32–6.

Income Data Services (1998) *Pay and Conditions in Call Centres 1998*, London: IDS.

Independent Television Commission (1998) 'ITC Notes: No 25, Sport on Television'. Available HTTP: http://www.itc.org.uk/ (25 November 1999).

– (1999) 'Television Audience Share Figures'. Online. Available HTTP: http://www.itc.org.uk/ (25 November 1999)

International Labour Office (ILO) (1998) 'Employability in the global economy: how training matters', *World Employment Report 1998–9*, Geneva: ILO.

Internet Society (1999) Online. Available HTTP: http://www.isoc.org (20 October 1999).

Internet Software Consortium (1999) *Internet Domain Survey*. Online. Available HTTP: http://www.isc.org/ds (20 October 1999).

Jenson, J., Hagen, E. and Reddy, C. (eds) (1988) *The Feminisation of the Labour Force*, Cambridge: Polity.

Johnson, E. (1956) *The Community Education Project: A Four Year Report 1952–6*. San Bernadino, CA: San Bernadino Valley College.

Jordan, T. (1999) *Cyberpower, The Culture and Politics of Cyberspace and the Internet*, London: Routledge.

Karpf, A. (1987) 'Recent feminist approaches to women and technology', in M. McNeil (ed.) *Gender and Expertise*, London: Free Association Books.

Katz, J. E. and Aspden, P. (1998) 'Internet dropouts in the USA', *Telecommunications Policy* 22, 4/5: 327–39.

Keane, J. (1991) *The Media and Democracy*, Cambridge: Polity.

– 1992, 'Democracy and the media – without foundations', *Political Studies* 40: 116–29.

Keynes, J. M. (1930) *A Treatise on Money*, London: Macmillan.

Kumar, K. (1986) 'Public service broadcasting and the public interest', in C. MacCabe and O. Stewart (eds) *The BBC and Public Service Broadcasting*, Manchester: Manchester University Press.

– (1995) *From Post-Industrial to Post-Modern Society*, London: Blackwell.
– (1997) *Rebuilding Societies After Civil War: Critical Roles For International Assistance*, Boulder: Lynne Rienner.
Kuznets, S. (1955) 'Economic growth and income inequality', *American Economic Review*, 45,1: 1–28.
Kvande, E. and Ramussen, B. (1989) 'Men, women and data systems', *European Journal of Engineering Education* 14,4: 369–79
Lappé, F. M. (1985) *Diet for a Small Planet*, New York: Ballantine.
Lange, A. and Renaud, J. (1989) *The Future of the European Audio-Visual Industry*, Manchester: European Institute for the Media.
Langham, D. (1994) 'Preserving Democracy in Cyberspace: the need for a new literacy', *Computer-Mediated Communication* 1, 4:7 Online. Available HTTP: http://metalab.unc.edu/cmc/mag/1994/aug/literacy.html (10 May 1998)
Layng, Sanderson and Associates (1989) *1988 Community Channel Survey*, Ottawa CRTC.
Leggewie, C. (1997) 'Netizens: Another structural change of the public sphere? Prospects for democratic participation in the Internet,' *IWM Working Papers 1*. Online. Available HTTP: http://www.univie.ac.at/iwm/workpap/leggewie.html (10 May 1998).
Lewis, C. (1924) *Broadcasting from Within*, London: George Newnes.
Lewis, P. (1978) *Whose Media? The Annan Report: A Citizen's Guide to Radio and Television*, London: Consumers' Association.
Linn, P. (1987) 'Gender stereotypes, technology stereotypes', in M. McNeil (ed.) *Gender and Expertise*, London: Free Association Books.
Livingstone, S. and Lunt, P. (1994) *Talk on Television: Audience Participation and Public Debate*, London: Routledge.
Loader, B.D. (ed.) (1998) *Cyberspace Divide. Equality, Agency and Policy in the Information Society*, London: Routledge.
Lundvall, B.A. (1998) 'The globalising learning economy: implications for small and medium sized enterprises', mimeo, Department of Business Studies, Aalborg University.
Lyon, D. (1988) *The Information Society, Issues and Illusions*, Cambridge: Polity.
Lyotard, J.-F. (1984), *The Postmodern Condition: A Report of Knowledge*, trans. G. Bennington and B. Massumi, Minneapolis: University of Minnesota Press.
McChesney, R. (1996) 'The Internet and U.S. Communication Policy-Making in Historical and Critical Perspective' in *Journal of Communication* 46 (1), Winter 1996, 98–124.
McIntosh, N. (1999) 'The new poor', *The Guardian* (22 July).
MacKenzie, D. and Wajcman, J. (eds) (1985) *The Social Shaping of Technology*, Milton Keynes: Open University Press.
McNeil, M. (1987) 'It's a man's world', in M. McNeil (ed.) *Gender and Expertise*, London: Free Association Books.
McNulty, J. (1988) 'Technology and nation-building in Canadian broadcasting', in R. Lorimer and R. Wilson (eds) *Communications Canada: Issues in Broadcasting and New Technologies*, Toronto: Kagan and Woo.

McQuail, D. and the Euromedia Research Group (1990) 'Caging the beast: constructing a framework for the analysis of media change in western Europe', *European Journal of Communication* 5: 313–31.

Maddison A. (1991) *Dynamic Forces in Capitalist Development: A Long-Run Comparative View*, Oxford: Oxford University Press.

Mahoney, P. and van Toen, B. (1990) 'Mathematical formalism as a means of occupational closure in computing: why hard computing tends to exclude women', *Gender and Education* 2,3: 319–31.

Maslow, A.H. (1962) *Toward a Psychology of Being*, Princeton: Van Nostrand.

Massey, D. (1988) 'What's happening to UK manufacturing?' in A. Allen and D. Massey (eds) (1988) *The Economy in Question*, London: Sage.

Masuda, Y. (1985) 'Computopia', in T. Forester (ed.) *The Information Technology Revolution*, Oxford: Basil Blackwell.

Mattelart, A. and Piemme, J.-M. (1980) 'New means of communication: new questions for the left', *Media, Culture and Society* 2,4: 321–39.

Mihill, C. (1998) 'Drug firm donates £1 billion to defeat tropical disease', *The Guardian* (27 January).

Milkman, R. (1998) 'The new American workplace: high road or low road?', in P. Thompson and C. Warhurst (eds) *Workplaces of the Future*, London: MacMillan.

Mill, J. (1820/1967) *Essays on Government, Jurisprudence and the Law of Nations* (reprint). New York, NY:Kelley.

Millar, J. (1998) 'International software trade: managing knowledge sharing between developing country producers and their clients', mimeo, SPRU, University of Sussex.

Miller, N., Leung, L. and Kennedy, H. (1997) 'Challenging boundaries in adult and higher education through technological innovation', in P. Armstrong, N. Miller and M. Zukas (eds) *Crossing Borders, Breaking Boundaries: Research in the Education of Adults*, London: SCUTREA.

Mitter, S. (1986) *Common Fate, Common Bond. Women in the Global Economy*, London: Pluto.

Morris, M. and Ogan, C. (1996) 'The Internet as mass medium', *Journal of Communication*, 46,1: 39–50.

Mumford, L. (1967) *The Myth of the Machine, vol. 1: Technics and Human Development*, New York: Harcourt Brace Jovanovich.

NOP (1999) *Internet User Profile Study*, London: National Opinion Polls.

NTIA (1998) 'Falling Through the Net II: new data on the digital divide'. National Telecommunications and Information Administration (NTIA). Online. Available HTTP: http://www.ntia.doc.gov/ntiahome/net2/falling.html (19 October 1999).

– (1999a) 'Falling Through the Net III: defining the digital divide'. NTIA. Online. Available HTTP: http://www.ntia.doc.gov/ntiahome/fttn99/contents.html (19 October 1999).

– (1999b) 'Internet Domain Names: Papers and Comments'. NTIA. Online. Available HTTP: http://www.ntia.doc.gov/ntiahome/domainname/domainhome.html (19 October 1999).

Naisbitt, J. (1984) *Megatrends: Ten New Directions Transforming Our Lives*, New York: Warner Books.

Negrine, R. (1988) 'New media in Britain: is there a policy?' in K. Dyson, P. Humphries with R. Negrine and J.P. Simon (eds) *Broadcasting and New Media Policies in Western Europe*, London: Routledge.

– (1989) *Politics and the Mass Media in Britain*, London: Routledge.

Negroponte, N. (1995) *Being Digital*, London: Hodder & Stoughton.

Negt, O. (1978) 'Mass media: tools of domination or instruments of liberation? Aspects of the Frankfurt School's communications analysis', *New German Critique* 14: 61–80.

Newham Online (1999) Online. Available HTTP: http://www.newham.org.uk (20 October 1999).

Noam, E. M. (1994) 'Beyond Liberalisation III: reforming universal service', *Telecommunications Policy* 18,9: 687–704.

OECD (McCracken Report) (1977) *Towards Full Employment and Price Stability*, Paris: Organisation for Economic Co-operation and Development (OECD).

– (1993) *Employment Outlook*, Paris: OECD.

– (1994) *The OECD Jobs Study – Facts, Analysis, Strategy*, Paris: OECD.

– (1997) 'New Directions for Industrial Policy', *Policy Brief 3*, Paris: OECD.

– (1998) *The Multinational Agreement on Investment, The MAI Negotiating Text (as of 14 February)*, Paris: OECD.

OFTEL (1999) 'Universal Telecommunication Services: a consultative document issued by the Director General of Telecommunications'. Online. Available HTTP: http://www.oftel.gov.uk/consumer/uts799.htm (20 October 1999).

O'Malley, T. (1994) *Closedown? The BBC and Government Broadcasting Policy, 1979–1992*, London: Pluto.

O'Reilly J. (1994) *Banking on Flexibility*, Aldershot: Avebury.

Pakulski, J. and Waters, M. (1996) *The Death of Class*, London: Sage.

Patient, S. (1999) 'A right royal question (free vs. paid-for Internet access)', *Internet Magazine* 58, September: 34–40.

Payne R. (1998) *The Hidden Call Centre Opportunity*, Bussum: Versatility.

Perez, C. (1983) 'Structural change and the assimilation of new technologies in the economic and social system', *Futures* 15,5: 357–75.

– (1998) 'Technological revolutions and the changing relationship between financial and productive capital', paper presented at 'Production Capitalism vs. Financial Capitalism: An Evolutionary Perspective' conference, Oslo.

Phillips, A. and Taylor, B. (1986) 'Sex and skill: notes towards a feminist economics', in Feminist Review (eds) *Waged Work: a Reader*, London: Virago.

Pimlott, H. (1992) '(Un)Limited horizons?: Canadian community television and the extension of the public sphere', unpublished M.A. dissertation, Goldsmiths College, University of London.

Pinch, T. and Bijker, W. (1987) 'The social construction of facts and artifacts: or how the sociology of science and the sociology of technology might benefit each other', in W. Bijker, T. Hughes and T. Pinch (eds) *The Social Construction of Technological Systems*, Cambridge, MA: MIT Press.

Poster, M. (1995) 'The net as a public sphere?', *Wired* March. Online. Available HTTP: http://vip.hotwired.com/wired/3.11/departments/poster.if.html (10 May 1998).

Poynter, G. (2000) *Restructuring in the Services Industries: Management Reform and Workplace Relations in the UK Service Sector*, London: Cassell.

Pritchett, L. (1995) 'Divergence big time', *Policy Research Working Paper 1522*, Washington: World Bank.

PTTI (Postal, Telegraph and Telephone International) (1998) *Downsizing, Contracting Out and New Opportunities for Telephone Operators Jobs*, Geneva: PTTI.

Quinn J. and Gagnon C. (1985) 'Will services follow manufacturing into decline?' *Harvard Business Review* November-December: 95–103.

Rajan, A. (1984) *New Technology and Employment in Insurance, Banking and Building Societies*, Aldershot: Gower.

Rheingold, H. (1991) 'The great equalizer', *Whole Earth Review* Summer: 6.

– (1994) *The Virtual Community: Finding Connection in a Computerized World*, London: Secker & Warburg.

Robins, K. and Webster, F. (1987) 'Information as capital: a critique of Daniel Bell', in J. Slack and F. Fejes (eds) *The Ideology of the Information Age*, Norwood: Ablex Publishing Corporation.

Robins, K and Webster, F. (1989) *The Technical Fix: Education, Computers and Industry*, London: Macmillan.

Rowan, D. (1998) 'Meet the new world government', *The Guardian* (13 February).

Sachs, J. D. (1997) 'IMF orthodoxy isn't what Southeast Asia needs', *International Herald Tribune* (4 November).

– (1998) 'Out of the frying pan into the IMF fire', *Observer* (8 February).

Salter, L. (1988) 'Reconceptualizing public broadcasting', in R. Lorimer and R. Wilson (eds) *Communications Canada: Issues in Broadcasting and New Technologies*, Toronto: Kagan and Woo.

Sayer, A. and Walker, R. (1992) *The New Social Economy*, Oxford: Blackwell.

Scannell, P. (1990) 'Public service broadcasting: the history of a concept', in A. Goodwin and G. Whannel (eds) *Understanding Television*, London: Routledge.

Schumpeter, J. A. (1939) *Business Cycles* (2 vols), New York: McGraw Hill.

Sears, T. (1991) 'Encouraging women returners into computing courses in higher education', in G. Lovegrove and B. Segal (eds) *Women into Computing: Selected Papers 1988–1990*, Amsterdam: Springer Verlag.

Sen, A. (1992) *Inequality Re-examined*, Oxford: Oxford University Press.

– (1999) 'Assessing Human Development' in UNDP, *Human Development Report, 1999*, Oxford: Oxford University Press.

Senker, J. (1999) 'Biotechnology: Scientific progress and social progress', paper for *Biotecnologia, Industria y Sociedad (BIOSPAIN 99)*, Valencia.

Senker, P. (1989) 'Managers, technology and market forces', *Journal of General Management* 15,1: 4–18.

– (1995) 'Technological change and the future of work', in N. Heap, R. Thomas, G. Einon, R. Mason and H. Mackay (eds) *Information Technology and Society*, London: Sage.

Shamberg, M. (1971) *Guerrilla Television*, New York: Holt Rinehart & Winston.

Shiva, V. (1997) Biodiversity totalitarianism – IPRs as seed monopolies, *Economic and Political Weekly*, 32,41: 2582–5.

Siann, G. (1997) 'We can, we don't want to: factors influencing women's participation in computing', in R. Lander and A. Adam (eds) *Women in Computing*, Exeter: Intellect Books.

Siepmann, C. (1952) *Television and Education in the United States*, New York: UNESCO.

Siune, K. and Truetzschler, W. (1992) 'Television Content: Dallasification of Culture', in K. Siune and W. Truetzschler for the Euromedia Research Group (eds) *Dynamics of Media Politics: Broadcast and Electronic Media in Western Europe*, London: Sage.

Smith, A. (1776/1974) *The Wealth of Nations*, London: Pelican.

Smith, A. (1986) 'Licences and liberty: public service broadcasting in Britain', in C. MacCabe and O. Stewart (eds) *The BBC and Public Service Broadcasting*, Manchester: Manchester University Press.

Spender, D. (1996) *Nattering on the Net: Women, Power and Cyberspace*, North Melbourne: Spinifex Publishing.

Stepulevage, L. (1997) 'Sexuality and computing: transparent relations', in G. Griffin and S. Andermahr (eds) *Straight Studies Modified: Lesbian Interventions in the Academy*, London: Cassell.

Stepulevage, L. and Plumeridge, S. (1996) 'Deconstruction of computer science as science' *Innovation Studies Working Paper No.11*, London: Department of Innovation Studies, University of East London.

– (1998) 'Women taking positions within computer science', *Gender and Education* 10,3: 313–26

Stocks, M. (1949) *Eleanor Rathbone, A Biography*, London: Gollancz.

Stonier T. (1983) *The Wealth of Information: A Profile of the Post-Industrial Economy*, London: Thames Methuen.

Surman, M. (1997) *From VTR to Cyberspace: Jefferson, Gramsci & the Electronic Commons*. Online. Available HTTP: http://kows.web.net/ecommons/gramsci/html (6 March 1997).

Tawney, R. H. (1964) *Inequality*, London: Unwin (first published in 1931).

Taylor P. (1998) 'Emotional labour and the new workplace' in P. Thompson and C. Warhurst (eds) *Workplaces of the Future*, London: MacMillan.

Technology Assessment and Forecast (TAF) Branch, US Patent and Trademark Office (1999) *General Statistical Reports*, Washington, DC: USPTO.

Thomas, G. and Wyatt, S. (1999) 'Shaping cyberspace – interpreting and transforming the Internet', *Research Policy*, 28,7: 681–98.

Thompson, P. and Warhurst, C. (eds) (1998) *Workplaces of the Future*, London: MacMillan.

Thrupp, L.A. (1996) 'Overview', in L.A. Thrupp (ed.) *New Partnerships for Sustainable Agriculture*, Washington: World Resources Institute.

de Tocqueville, A. (1839/1963) *Democracy in America*, Oxford: Oxford's World Classics.

Toffler, A. (1980) *The Third Wave*, London: Collins.

Turkle, S. (1995) *Life on the Screen: Identity in the Age of the Internet*, New York: Simon & Schuster.

Trudel, L. (1991) 'Alternative television: from myth to reality', in N. Thede and A. Ambrosi (eds) *Video the Changing World*, Montreal: Black Rose Books.

Tuer, D. (1994) 'All in the family: an examination of community access cable in Canada', *Fuse* 18,1: 23–31.

UNDP (United Nations Development Programme) (1997) *Human Development Report, 1997*, New York: Oxford University Press.

– (1999) *Human Development Report*, New York: Oxford University Press. Online. Available HTTP: http://www.undp.org/hdro/report.html (19 October 1999).

van Oost, E. (1992) 'The masculinisation of the computer: a historical reconstruction', paper presented at 'Gender, Technology and Ethics' conference, Lund.

van Zoonen, L. (1992) 'Feminist theory and information technology', *Media, Culture and Society* 14: 9–29.

Veljanowski, C. (1989) *Freedom in Broadcasting*, London: Institute of Economic Affairs.

Verne, G. (1991) 'Women's challenge to computer science and technology', *International Journal of Science Education* 9,3: 361–6.

Vidal, J. (1997) 'Empire of burgers' *The Guardian* (20 June).

Wade, R. (1990) *Governing the Market: Economic Theory and the Role of Government in East Asian Industrialisation*, Princeton: Princeton University Press.

Walkerdine, V. (1989) *Counting Girls Out*, London: Virago.

Warhurst, C. and Thompson, P. (1998) 'Hands, hearts and minds: changing work and workers at the end of the century', in P. Thompson and C. Warhurst (eds) *Workplaces of the Future*, London: Macmillan.

Waters, M. (1995) *Globalization*, Routledge, London.

Watkins, K. (1997) 'The free way to poverty', *The Guardian* (5 February).

Webster, F. (1995) *Theories of the Information Society*, London: Routledge.

Whiston, T.G. (1993) 'Prospects for the 21st century – the global challenge: tasks for the 21st century', *Outlook on Agriculture* 22,4: 252–6.

Williamson, J.G. and Lindert, P. H. (1980) *American Inequality: A Macroeconomic History*, New York: Academic Press.

Winston, B. (1998) *Media Technology and Society. A History: From the Telegraph to the Internet*, London: Routledge.

Wolfensohn, J. (1998) 'Asia, the long view', *Financial Times* (29 January).

World Bank (1991) *World Development Report 1991*, New York: Oxford University Press.

Wyatt, S. (1998) *Technology's Arrow, Developing Information Networks for Public Administration in Britain and the United States*, Maastricht: Universitaire Pers Maastricht.

Zakon, R.H. (1999) *Hobbes Internet Timeline*. Online. Available HTTP: http://www.isoc.org/zakon/Internet/History/HIT.html (19 October 1999).

Zuboff , S. (1988) *In the Age of the Smart Machine: The Future of Work and Power*, Oxford: Heinneman.

INDEX

Ellul, J. 18
employment 5, 13, 17, 69, 74, 118, 143, 155–6, 158–63, 172, 175, 177–83, 189, 194–6, 200–2, 204–5; see also unemployment
Enzensberger, H.M. 89
encryption 38, 42, 72–3, 76, 81
equality see inequality
Ess, C. 57
Euromedia Research Group 80–1
Europe 28, 33, 49, 62, 64, 74–8, 82, 106, 150, 154, 160, 178, 184–5, 190, 198, 200–1, 203, 213
European Parliament 43
European Commission 69, 75–8, 83–4, 200–1, 204
Evening Standard, The 81

Fagerberg, J. 203
Farago, R. 192
Federal Communications Commission (FCC) 49, 54
feminism 114, 118
Ferry, J. 76
Finch, J. 210–11
Fincham, R. 176, 181, 192–3, 195
Fisher, A. 177
Fisher, I. 159
flexibility: broadcasting 75, 81; design 34, 43; education 133–4, 136–8, 142–3; workplace 184, 189–90, 196
football 33, 55, 61–2, 82, 85
Ford, H. 159
Ford Motor Company163
France 49, 92, 106, 163, 185
Franks, S. 70, 82
Freeman, C. 8, 12, 17, 149
Fryer Report 59, 133–5, 138

Gagnon, C. 180
Galbraith, J.K. 159
Gallie, D. 174
Game, A. 114
Garnham, N. 56, 64–8, 75, 78, 84
Gaynor, D. 57
genetic modification 202, 207, 209, 215–16

Georgia Technical University (Internet user survey) 27
Germany 49, 92, 106
Gershuny, J. 13
Giddens, A. 7
Gill, R. 113
Gillespie, G. 107
globalisation 80, 169, 205, 213
Goldberg, K. 98, 101, 107
Golding, P. 63
government 13, 15–16, 25, 42–3, 47, 52, 57, 59–60, 65, 68–71, 74–5, 82, 86, 88–9, 92, 132, 135, 151–3, 163, 167, 171, 185, 201–4, 206–8, 214; Canadian 86, 95–8, 100, 104–5, 107; French 83; New Labour 133, 136, 216; US 22
Green, E. 15
Green, J. 192
Greenpeace 216
Greenspan, A. 159
Gregory, A. 182
Grint, K. 113
Groombridge, B. 48, 50–1
Grossman, L. 57
Guardian Royal Exchange 193
Guardian, The 1

Habermas, J. 56–8, 67, 92–3, 100, 106–7
Hacker, S. 114
Hafner, K. 44
Hall, P. 131
Hamel, G. 172
Hammer, M. 180, 190
Hammersley, B. 61
Handy, C. 174
Haraway, D. 14
Hardin, H. 97–8, 107
have-nots 1, 2, 4, 42, 87, 161; see also inequality
Hayes, D. 84
Haywood, T. 15
Head, S. 180
Henderson, J. 178
Henwood, F. 8, 12, 17, 113–14, 127
heterosexuality 127 see also lesbians and gays